Manual of Psychiatric
Nursing Care Plans

Manual of Psychiatric Nursing Care Plans

Judith M. Schultz, B.A., R.N., B.S.N.
University of Missouri School of Nursing,
Columbia, Missouri

Sheila L. Dark, R.N., B.S.N.
Allen Memorial Hospital Lutheran School
of Nursing, Waterloo, Iowa

Little, Brown and Company, Boston

Contents

Preface

The *Manual of Psychiatric Nursing Care Plans* was conceived as and written to be a reference manual—a practical guide to nursing care planning based on the behaviors of clients commonly encountered in nursing practice, particularly in mental health nursing. It has been designed to facilitate implementation of the nursing process for clients with emotional problems.

Each client is an individual and therefore needs a plan of nursing care specifically tailored to his or her own needs, problems, and circumstances. These care plans do not replace the nurse's skills in assessment, problem identification, goal setting, implementation, and evaluation of nursing care. Rather, the plans contain a range of emotional and behavioral problems that may be encountered and a variety of approaches that may be employed. This information must be adapted and used as appropriate in the nurse's planning of care for each individual client.

This book, then, is not intended to replace individual care planning, nor is it offered as a complete psychiatric nursing text. It is a resource, a learning tool, and a reference book that presents information, concepts, and principles in a simple and clear format so the nurse can use it in a variety of settings and situations. Because the *Manual* offers concrete suggestions for particular situations and can be adapted to the care of any client, it will be helpful in both academic and clinical settings.

The *Manual of Psychiatric Nursing Care Plans* is especially suited for use in classes in general and mental health nursing; in orientation and inservice programs in mental health, general medical, and continuing-care facilities; and in continuing education programs for practicing nurses. It is ideal as a handbook in both mental health and general medical units for use in developing individual care plans and in helping new staff members by offering clear and specific approaches to various problems. It can be used also by non-professional health care staff members and non-nursing staff members, and can be especially helpful in the general medical or continuing-care facility, where staff members may encounter these kinds of behaviors infrequently and may have less formal education and less self-confidence in dealing with clients who are experiencing emotional difficulties.

We believe that effective nursing care must begin with a holistic view of each client, whose life includes a particular complex of physical, emotional, spiritual, interpersonal, and socioeconomic factors. We sincerely hope that the *Manual of Psychiatric Nursing Care Plans* contributes to that nursing care process.

J. M. S.
S. L. D.

Acknowledgments

The writing of a book always involves many more people than the authors alone, and we wish to express our thanks to those most involved in this process. Primarily, we acknowledge our gratitude to all the clients (and their families or significant others) with whom we have worked. They have not only taught us about human behavior but have also enriched our lives by sharing theirs with us. Also, this book had its beginning in the Mid-Missouri Mental Health Center, Columbia, Missouri, and thanks are due to Carol Spengler, R.N., M.S.; to the Departments of Nursing and Nursing Education for providing a supportive environment; to the staff members of Unit 2-Center (in the mid-1970s) whose ideas were included in some of the early versions of these care plans, especially Luke Lundemo and John Esterly; and to the early members of the committee on developing standardized care plans: Sharon Hyler, R.N., Mary Kennish, R.N., Sharon Lavery, R.N., Kathy Meyers, R.N., and the late Mary Dell Craft, R.N.

Thanks, too, to Guyla Stidmon for both the typing of the manuscript and her steadfastness over a number of years. We also thank Little, Brown and Company for their support, encouragement, and patience, and especially Ann West, Nursing Developmental Editor.

Finally, in the personal realm, our heartfelt thanks to our parents, who helped make our education possible, and to Hank Dark and Linda Delano for their continuing support, ideas, insights, and feedback throughout this endeavor.

Manual of Psychiatric
Nursing Care Plans

BASIC CONCEPTS

I

The care plans in this book have been created with certain fundamental concepts in mind as premises upon which the plans were built. In this section, we will delineate these concepts and beliefs, hoping to stimulate the reader's thinking about these aspects of working with clients.

FUNDAMENTAL BELIEFS

1. A nurse provides only what care the client cannot provide for himself or herself at the time.
2. The client is at all times responsible for his or her own feelings, actions, and life (see "Client Responsibilities" below).
3. The client must be approached by the nurse as a whole person with a unique background, environment, strengths, and set of behaviors or problems, not as a psychiatrically labeled nonentity to be manipulated.
4. The client is not a passive recipient of care. The nurse and the client work together toward goals that have been mutually determined as desirable. The client's active participation in all steps in the nursing process should be encouraged within the limits of the client's present level of functioning (see "Client Responsibilities").
5. The predominant focus of work with the client is health, not merely absence or diminution of the disease process. This means, too, that one goal of therapy is the client's eventual independence from the hospital and staff. If this is impossible, then the client should reach his or her optimum level of functioning and independence.
6. Given feedback and the identification of alternative ways to meet needs (acceptable to the client), the client will generally opt to progress toward a more healthful lifestyle with appropriate coping mechanisms.
7. Physical and emotional health are interconnected; therefore, physical health is a desirable goal in the treatment of emotional problems. Nursing care should incorporate this concept and focus on the client's obtaining adequate nutrition, rest, and exercise, and the elimination of substance abuse (including tobacco, caffeine, alcohol, over-the-counter medications, or other drugs) as part of the client's progress toward health.
8. The nurse works with other health professionals (and nonprofessionals) in a multidisciplinary approach within a milieu that is constructed as a therapeutic environment. The nurse may function as team coordinator with the aim of developing a holistic view of the client.

THERAPEUTIC MILIEU

Purpose and Definition

The therapeutic milieu is an environment that is structured and maintained as an ideal, dynamic setting in which to work with clients. This milieu includes safe physical surroundings, all staff members, and other clients. A therapeutic setting should minimize environmental stress, such as noise and confusion, and physical stress caused by such factors as substance abuse or lack of sleep.

Removal of the client from a stressful environment to a therapeutic environment provides a chance for rest and nurturance of self, a time to focus on the development of strengths, and an opportunity to learn to identify alternatives or solutions to problems and the psychodynamics of

1

those problems. This setting also allows clients to take part in a community in which they can share feelings and experiences and enjoy social interaction and growth as well as "therapy." The nurse has a unique opportunity to facilitate (and model) communication and sharing among clients in the creation of continuing, dynamic, informal group therapy.

A therapeutic milieu is a "safe space," a nonpunitive atmosphere in which caring is a given. In this environment, confrontation may be a positive therapeutic tool that can be tolerated by the client. Nurses and other staff members should be aware of their own roles in this environment, minimizing an authoritarian position (e.g., displaying keys as a reminder of status), yet maintaining a professional role (see "Nursing Responsibilities" below). Clients are expected to assume responsibility for themselves within the unit structure when they are ready to do so. Feedback from other clients and the sharing of duties facilitate the client's growth.

Maintaining a Safe Environment

One important aspect of a therapeutic environment is the exclusion of objects or circumstances that may be used by a client to harm self or others. Although this is especially important in a mental health care setting, this should be considered in any health care situation.

The nursing staff should follow the facility's policies with regard to prevention of routine safety hazards and supplement these policies as necessary, for example:

Dispose of all needles safely and out of reach of clients.
Restrict or monitor use of matches and lighters.
Do not allow smoking in bedrooms (clients may be drowsy due to the use of psychotropic drugs).
Remove mouthwash, cologne, aftershave, and so forth if substance abuse is suspected.

Listed below are the most restrictive measures to be used with clients who are exhibiting behavior directly threatening or harmful to self or others. These measures may be modified on the basis of the assessment of the client's behavior.

Do not use glass containers (ashtrays, drinking glasses, vases, salt and pepper shakers).

Be sure mirrors, if glass, are securely fastened.
Keep sharp objects (scissors, pocket knives, knitting needles) out of reach of clients and allow their use only with supervision.
Use electric shavers when possible (disposable razors are easily broken and blades removed).
Identify potential weapons (mop handles, hammers, pool cues, baseball bats) and dangerous equipment (electrical cords, scalpels, pap smear fixative); keep out of clients' reach.
Do not leave cleaning or maintenance carts (cleaning fluids, bleach, mops, tools) unattended in client-care areas.
Do not leave medicines unattended or unlocked.
Keep keys (to unit door, medicines) on person at all times.
Be aware of items which are harmful if ingested, e.g., poisonous plants (philodendron), thermometers.

Immediately upon the client's admission to the facility, staff members should search the client and all of the client's belongings and remove potentially dangerous items such as wire hangers, ropes, belts, safety pins, scissors and other sharp objects, weapons, and medications. Keep these belongings in a designated place inaccessible to the client. Also, search any packages brought by visitors (it may be necessary to search visitors in certain circumstances). Explain the reason for such rules briefly, and do not make exceptions.

The Trust Relationship

One of the keys to a therapeutic environment is the establishment of trust. Not only must the client come to trust the nurse, but also the nurse must trust himself or herself as a therapist, must trust in the client's motivation and ability to change, and both the client and the nurse must trust that therapy is desirable and productive.

Trust is the foundation of a therapeutic relationship, and consistency and limit-setting are the building blocks. A trust relationship between the nurse and the client creates a space in which they can work together using the nursing process and their best possible efforts toward goals they have both identified. (See Care Plan 1, Building a Trust Relationship.)

Building Self-Esteem

Just as a physically healthy body may be better able to withstand stress, a person with adequate or high self-esteem may be better able to deal with emotional difficulties. Thus, an essential part of a client's care is helping to build the client's self-esteem.

Since each client retains the responsibility for his or her own feelings, and one person cannot *make* another person feel a certain way, the nurse cannot increase the client's self-esteem directly. Strategies to help build or enhance self-esteem must be individualized. Some general suggestions are:

Build a trust relationship with the client (see Care Plan 1, Building a Trust Relationship).

Set and maintain limits (see "Limit-Setting" below).

Accept the client as a person.

Be nonjudgmental at all times.

Provide structure (structure the client's time and activities).

Have realistic expectations of the client.

Make your expectations clear to the client.

Provide the client with tasks, responsibilities, and activities that can be easily accomplished; advance the client to more difficult tasks as he or she progresses.

Praise the client for his or her accomplishments, however small, giving sincere appropriate feedback for meeting expectations, completing tasks, fulfilling responsibilities, and so on.

Never flatter the client or be otherwise dishonest.

Minimize negative feedback to the client without giving mixed messages (e.g., enforce the limits that have been set, but withdraw attention if possible rather than chastising the client for exceeding limits).

Use confrontation judiciously and in a supportive manner; use it only when the client can tolerate it.

Allow the client to make his or her own decisions whenever possible.

Limit-Setting

Integral to a trust relationship and to a therapeutic milieu are the setting and maintaining of limits. Effective limits can provide a structure and a sense of caring that words alone cannot, and will also minimize manipulation and secondary gains in therapy.

First, state the expectation or the limit as clearly, directly, and simply as possible. The consequence that will follow the client's exceeding the limit must also be clearly stated at the outset. Before stating the limit and consequence, you may wish to go over briefly with the client the reasons for limit-setting, and involve the client in this part of care planning; together you may decide on specific limits or consequences. However, if this is impossible, briefly explain the limits to the client, and do not indulge in lengthy discussions or give undue attention to the consequences of infraction of a limit.

Second, keep in mind that consequences should be direct, simple, have some bearing on the limit if possible, and be something that the client perceives as a negative outcome, not as a reward or producer of secondary gain. For example, if the consequence is not allowing the client to go to an activity, it will not be effective if (a) the client did not want to go anyway; (b) the client is allowed to watch television instead, which the client may prefer; or (c) the client receives individual attention from the staff at that time, which the client may prefer.

Third, the consequence should immediately follow the client's exceeding the limit and must be consistent, both over time (each time the limit is exceeded) and among the staff (each staff member must enforce the limit). One staff person may be designated to make decisions regarding the client and limits to ensure consistency; however, when this person is not available, another person must take that responsibility rather than defer the consequences.

Remember, although consequences are essential to setting and maintaining limits, they are *not* an opportunity to be punitive to a client. The withdrawal of attention is perhaps the best and simplest of consequences to carry out, provided that attention and support are given when the client meets expectations and remains within limits. If the only time the client receives attention and feedback, albeit negative, is when he or she exceeds limits, that client will continue to elicit attention in that way. The client must perceive a positive reason to meet expectations; there must be a reward for staying within limits.

Remember, too, that a client does not need the nurse as a friend or a sympathetic person who will be "nice." By allowing a client to exceed limits, you will be giving the client mixed messages and will undermine the other staff members as well as the client. You will convey to the client that you do not in fact care enough for the client's growth and well-being to enforce a limit, and you will betray a lack of control on your part at a time when the client feels out of control and expressly needs someone else to be in control. (See "Nursing Responsibilities" below; Care Plan 25, Passive-Aggressive or Manipulative Behavior, and Care Plan 26, Dependency or Inadequacy.)

Communication Techniques

Many communication techniques have been identified. The following have proved effective in fostering open communication with clients:

Offer yourself to the client for a specific period of time for the purpose of communication.

Talk about the client and the client's feelings, *not* about yourself, other clients, or the staff.

Allow the client enough time to talk.

Listen to the client; pay attention to what the client is saying, verbally and nonverbally.

Be comfortable using silence as a communication tool.

Make eye contact.

Ask open-ended questions. Avoid questions that can have one-word answers.

Encourage the client to ventilate feelings.

Be honest with the client.

Be nonjudgmental.

Know your own feelings and do not let them prejudice your interaction with the client.

Use the client's name and your name; the use of given names may be decided by the facility or the individual unit philosophies or may depend on the comfort of the client and the nurse or the nature of the client's problem.

Allow the client to explore alternatives; help the client to identify these.

Tell the client if you do not understand what he or she means; take the responsibility yourself for not understanding and ask the client to clarify, giving the client the responsibility for the explanation.

Give the client feedback based on your observations.

Reflect what the client is saying back to him or her. In simple reflection, repeat the client's statement with an upward inflection in your voice to indicate questioning. In more complex reflection, rephrase the client's statement to reflect the feeling the client is expressing; point out seemingly contradictory statements and ask for clarification. Avoid putting your words in the client's mouth—use such phrases as "I hear you saying. . . . Is that what you are feeling? Is that what you mean?"

Use humor judiciously, if at all. Never tease a client and remember that clients with certain problems will not understand abstractions such as humor.

Do not describe the client's feelings in your own words.

Do not use pat phrases or platitudes in response to the client's expression of feelings, thus cutting off the client or belittling the client's feelings.

Do not try to fool or manipulate the client.

Do not argue with the client or get involved in a power struggle.

Do not take the client's anger or negative expressions personally.

Do not give your personal opinions, beliefs, or experiences in relation to the client's problems.

Do not give advice or make decisions for the client. If you advise a client and your advice is "good" (that is, the proposed solution is successful), the client has not had the opportunity to problem-solve, to take responsibility or credit for a good decision, and to enjoy the increased self-esteem that comes from a successful action. If your advice is "bad," the client has missed a chance to learn from making a mistake, to experience that she or he can survive making a mistake, and has successfully evaded responsibility for making a decision. Instead, the client may blame the staff member or the hospital for whatever consequences ensue from that decision.

Expression of Feelings

A significant part of therapy is the client's expression of feelings. It is important for the nurse to encourage the client to ventilate feelings in ways that are nondestructive and acceptable to the client such as writing, talking, drawing, or physical activity. It may also be desirable to encourage expressions, such as crying, with which the client (or the nurse) may not feel entirely comfortable. The nurse can facilitate the expression of emotions by giving the client direct verbal support, by using silence, by handing the client tissues, and by allowing the client adequate time to ventilate (without probing for information or cutting off the client with pat remarks).

The goal in working with a client is not to avoid painful feelings, but to have the client express, discharge, and come to accept even "negative" emotions such as hatred, despair, and rage. In *accepting* the client's feelings, the nurse need not give *approval* to everything the client says. If you, the nurse, are uncomfortable with the client's ventilation of feelings, it is important that you examine your own feelings or talk with another staff member about them, and provide the client with a staff member who is more comfortable with those feelings. (See Care Plan 11, Grief Reaction, Care Plan 9, Depression, and Care Plan 1, Building a Trust Relationship.)

SEXUALITY

Another area in which staff members' feelings are often evoked and must be considered is that of human sexuality. Because it is basic to everyone, sexuality may be a factor with any client in a number of ways. First, the client may be charged with or convicted of a crime that is associated with sexual activity, such as incest, exhibitionism, or rape (see "Clients with Legal Problems"). Second, certain aspects of sexuality may be posing a problem for a client: the client may be impotent or experiencing menopause; the client may have been the victim of incest or rape; the client may feel guilty about masturbation or sexual activity outside of marriage; the client may be experiencing homosexual feelings, which are uncomfortable or unacceptable to him or her; or the client may be having difficulty adjusting to a change in sexual habits or feelings, such as first sexual activity, marriage, or the death or loss of a sexual partner. Third, the client may not feel that he or she has a problem with sexuality, but some aspect of the client's sexuality or lifestyle may be disturbing to the staff members, for example, sexual feelings or activity in the young or old client, homosexuality, or transvestism. Finally, sexual conversations or activity may occur on the unit, such as clients being sexual with one another, a client making sexual advances or displays to a staff member, or a client masturbating openly on the unit.

Problems related to sexual acting-out on the unit can be handled by setting and maintaining limits, again with an awareness of the nurse's own feelings (see "Limit-Setting" above).

The recognition and exploration of the staff member's own feelings about any of these situations is essential; too many times, feelings which are not acknowledged on a conscious level or expressed, even to oneself, influence the way the nurse relates to and cares for the client. In some instances, the nurse may find it necessary to withdraw from the client or the client's treatment because of the discomfort or conflict produced by such feelings. The important thing is to become and remain aware of your own feelings so as not to interfere with good nursing care for the client; awareness of your feelings can help you deal with them and the client appropriately. Adjustment problems can occur with a change in sexual feelings or activities or result from a difficult experience (e.g., being a victim of incest). These problems may be hard for a client to reveal initially or to share with more than one staff person or other clients. Be sensitive to the client's feelings in care planning (the client's participation may be helpful). A matter-of-fact approach on the part of the nurse can help to minimize the client's discomfort.

Homosexuality per se is no longer classified as a mental health disorder and, although a client may be a male homosexual or a lesbian, he or she may not feel that it is a problem. Indeed, many homosexual people feel positive about that aspect of their lives and have no desire to change. If a homosexual client seeks treatment for another problem (e.g., depression), do not assume that this problem is due to or even directly related to the client's homosexuality. Being a homosexual, however, can present a number of significant stresses to an individual, and these may or may not influence the client's problem. Aside from societal censure in general, the client faces possible loss of familial support, his or her job, housing, and children, by revealing his or her homosexuality. Even these stresses, however, must not be confused with the client's sexuality per se, and they should not be treated as sexual problems if the client does not identify them as such.

Sexual concerns may also conflict with the religious beliefs of both clients and staff members. It may be helpful to involve a chaplain or other clergy member in the client's treatment. Having respect for the client, examining the nurse's own feelings, maintaining a nonjudgmental attitude toward the client, encouraging expression of the client's feelings, and allowing the client to make his or her own decisions—these are the standards for working with clients in situations with a moral or religious dimension, whether the issue is abortion, celibacy, sterilization, impotence, transsexualism, or any other aspect of human sexuality.

ROLE OF THE PSYCHIATRIC NURSE

Nurse's Responsibilities and Functions

Within a health care facility and within a therapeutic relationship with a client, the nurse has certain responsibilities and functions. These include:

Recognizing and accepting the client as an individual

Client advocacy (see "Client Advocacy" below)

Assessing the client and planning nursing care (see "Nursing Process" below)

Involving the client and the client's significant others in all parts of the nursing process

Accepting the client's perceptions and expression of discomfort (do not require the client to prove distress or illness to you)

Providing a safe environment, including the protection of the client and others from injury (see "Safe Environment" above)

Providing external controls for the client until such time as the client can maintain self-control (see "Limit-Setting" above and Care Plan 24, Aggressive Behavior)

Providing a therapeutic environment (see "Therapeutic Milieu" above)

Examining and recognizing your own feelings and being willing to work through those feelings

Recognizing physical and emotional health as related and inseparable, with the aim of integrating physical and emotional nursing care

Identifying the client's optimum level of health and functioning, and making that level the goal of the nursing process

Cooperating with other professionals in various aspects of the client's care—coordination of a multi-disciplinary approach to care

Accurately observing and documenting the client's behavior

Providing safe nursing care, including medication administration and therapy: individual interactions (verbal and nonverbal), formal and informal group situations, activities, role-playing, etc.

Client teaching (see "Client Teaching" below)

Providing feedback to the client based on observations of the client's behavior

Maintaining honesty and a nonjudgmental attitude at all times

Maintaining a professional role with regard to the client (see "Professional Role" below)

Providing opportunities for the client to make his or her own decisions or mistakes and to assume responsibility for self, feelings, and life

Forming expectations of the client that are realistic and clearly stated

Continuing nursing education and the exploration of new ideas, theories, and research.

The Nursing Process

The nursing process is a dynamic and continuing activity, which includes:

1. assessment
2. identification of personal strengths and external resources
3. identification of goals and objectives
4. establishment of timing
5. identification of possible actions and solutions
6. evaluation
7. revision of all steps of the process.

Since every client is an individual in a unique situation, each care plan must be individualized. The care plans in this manual provide lists of possible behaviors and problems, goals, objectives, and actions, which may be incorporated into a client's individual care plan. (See Part II, Introduction to Care Plans.)

The first step in the nursing process, the assessment of the client, is crucial. In assessing a client in planning and implementing care in the area of mental health nursing, the following factors are important to consider:

1. Client participation. The client's perceptions should be elicited, as well as the client's expectations of hospitalization and staff. What would the client like to change? How can this happen?
2. Client's strengths. What are the client's strengths as perceived by the client and by the nurse?

3. Participation by client's family or significant others. How are other people's behaviors or problems affecting the client?
4. Transcultural considerations. What is the client's cultural background? In what kind of cultural environment is the client living (or was raised)?
5. Substance use or abuse. Consider the client's use of caffeine (symptoms of anxiety and high caffeine use are very similar), tobacco, alcohol, and illicit, prescription, and over-the-counter drugs (e.g., bromide poisoning can occur with abuse of some over-the-counter medications).
6. Reality orientation. Check for recent and remote memory as well as client's orientation to person, place, and time.
7. Allergies. It may be necessary to ask the client's significant others for reliable information or to check the client's past records if possible.
8. Complete physical systems review. Remember, the client may minimize, maximize, or be unaware of physical problems.
9. Dentures. These may be a factor in nutritional problems.
10. Prostheses. Does the client need assistance in ambulation or other activities of daily living?
11. Present medications.
12. Suicidal ideations. Has the client made suicide plans, gestures, or attempts, or does he or she have a history of suicidal behavior?
13. Presence of hallucinations or delusions.
14. Aggression. Does the client have a history or present problem of aggression toward others, homicidal thoughts or plans, or possession of weapons?
15. Family history. Have there been mental health problems in the client's family?
16. Living situation, job, relationships with others.
17. Sexuality. Are any aspects of sexuality causing problems for the client?
18. Activity level. What can the client do for himself or herself? What is psychomotor activity level? Does the client get regular exercise?
19. Eye contact. Does the client make eye contact with staff members or significant others? What is the frequency and duration of eye contact?
20. Affect and mood. Describe the client's general mood, facial expressions, and demeanor.
21. Ability to communicate. Include the nature and extent of both verbal and nonverbal communication. Does the client's significant other speak for him or her?
22. Tremors or fidgeting. Describe the nature, extent, and frequency of repetitive movements.
23. Daily living habits. What does the client do all day? How do the client's habits differ now from before the client's problems began?
24. Interests and hobbies. Include the client's hobbies both before the present problems began and those that continue to interest the client now.
25. Previous hospitalizations. Include both medical and psychiatric hospitalizations; note length of stay and reason for hospitalization.

Remember to assess the client in a holistic way, integrating any relevant information about the client's life, behavior, and feelings before implementing the nursing process. Also remember that the focus of care, beginning with the initial assessment, is toward the client's optimum level of health and independence from the hospital.

Professional Role

Maintaining a professional role is essential in working with clients. A client comes to a health care facility for help, not to engage in social relationships or interactions. The client needs a nurse, not a friend: it is neither necessary nor desirable for the client to like you personally in the therapeutic situation.

Because the therapeutic milieu is not a social environment, the nurse must not offer personal information or beliefs to the client, or attempt to meet his or her own needs in the relationship. While this may seem severe, its importance extends beyond the establishment and maintenance of a therapeutic milieu. For example, a client who is considering abortion but who has not yet revealed this may ask the nurse if she or he is a Catholic. If the response is, "Yes," the client may assume that the nurse therefore is opposed to abortion and may be even more reluctant to discuss the problem. The point here is that the client must feel that the nurse, regardless of personal beliefs, will be accepting of him or her as a person and of the client's behaviors and problems. In addition, since a therapeutic relationship is not social, there is no reason for the nurse to discuss marital status, specific address, or phone number. If information of a personal nature such as this is requested by the client, it is appropriate for the nurse to respond by stating that such information is not necessary to the client and is inappropriate to the therapeutic relationship. The nurse can reinforce the principle of maintaining a therapeutic relationship as opposed to a social relationship at this time. Information of this nature might encourage a social relationship outside the hospital, dependence on a staff member after discharge, or it might endanger the nurse if the client is aggressive or hostile.

Staff Considerations

Much is said in this manual about the identification and expression of the feelings staff members have when working with clients. It will suffice here to state the importance of recognizing your own feelings and taking responsibility for them, because attempts to ignore such emotions often lead to a decreased awareness of the client's feelings and interference with the psychodynamics of the therapeutic interaction and with the honesty of the relationship as a whole.

A good way to increase awareness of staff feelings is to hold regular (though not necessarily rigidly scheduled or formal) client-care conferences and staff meetings. At least a part of these meetings can be devoted to the ventilation of feelings regarding clients. For example, staff members may be frustrated with a client who is not responding to treatment. At a client-care conference these feelings can be explored and the nursing care plan evaluated and revised, thus improving the client's care as well as preventing staff apathy and feelings of hopelessness regarding the client. Staff meetings can provide support for the feelings of staff members and provide the sense that a staff member is not alone in his or her reactions toward a client.

In addition to experiencing feelings of frustration and hopelessness, the staff may be uncomfortable with a client who is grieving, a homosexual client, a client who is considering abortion, or a client who is the perpetrator or the victim of a crime. Staff members may find themselves becoming angry with a client who is manipulative, hostile, or aggressive. A client's behavior may simply be difficult to tolerate or work with for extended periods of time (e.g., manic behavior). Then, the client-care conference can also be used to structure nursing care assignments to limit individual staff contacts with client to brief periods (e.g., 1 or 2 hours at a time). Remember, however, that expression of feelings is *not* passing judgment on the client or the client's behavior; it is done, rather, to avoid being judgmental or passive-aggressive in the client's care.

It is important in an acute situation to also identify your own emotions and deliberately withdraw from the client (if possible) if those feelings are interfering with your care of the client. If you find yourself reacting in an angry or punitive way, for example, it would be best to ask another staff member to deal with the client. In a therapeutic situation, the client's needs and well-being are paramount; it is the nurse's responsibility to remain in control (and to provide control for the client).

Client Advocacy

The nurse in the mental health care setting has a unique and vital role as a client advocate. Clients who are experiencing emotional problems are often unaware of their rights or unable to act in their own interest, and some clients (those hospitalized or restrained against their will) are almost completely dependent upon the staff to safeguard what rights are legally theirs. Also, the trauma and confusion of entering a mental health facility may be so overwhelming to the client and his or her family (or significant others) that they may become extremely passive in this regard. In addition to planning and implementing individualized nursing care in the best interest of the client, the nurse should be familiar with the rights of hospitalized clients in general and in specific cases (e.g., commitment) and monitor other aspects of client care with these in mind. The nurse can also identify herself or himself to the client as a client advocate and be available to help the client in this regard.

Client Teaching

Client teaching, like client advocacy, is an essential component of good nursing care. In the mental health field, health teaching may take many forms and may include giving information on topics such as the following:

General health: the relationship of physical and emotional health, nutrition, exercise, rest.

Emotional health: stress recognition and management, ways to increase emotional outlets, relaxation techniques.

Family and significant relationships: psychodynamics, secondary gains.

Medications: purpose, side effects (what to expect and how to minimize, if possible), special information (e.g., lithium carbonate blood level, toxicity).

Specific physical problems or continuing care: diabetes mellitus, how to change dressings, range of motion exercises.

Discharge planning: anticipating and planning for stresses or crises, identification of community resources for support after discharge, opportunity for continued therapy (group, outpatient) if necessary. (See Care Plan 2, Discharge Planning.)

ROLE OF THE CLIENT

Client's Responsibilities

A client who comes to a mental (or general) health care facility also has certain responsibilities within the therapeutic relationship. These include:

Recognizing and accepting his or her emotional problems

Recognizing and accepting that there is a relationship between physical and mental health

Recognizing and accepting hospitalization and/or treatment as positive steps toward the goal of optimum health

Recognizing and accepting the nurse as therapist

Accepting responsibility for his or her own feelings, even though that may be difficult or distasteful to the client's desired self-perception

Accepting an active role in his or her own treatment, being motivated toward achieving the goal of optimum health

Actively participating in care planning and implementation as soon and as much as possible.

Client's Rights

In mental health nursing, or any nursing practice in which mental health problems are encountered, the nurse must be aware of the state and federal laws regarding the clients' rights and certain aspects of client care. Anything that is deemed part of treatment but which is against the client's will must be examined by the nurse with respect to the law as well as to the client's well-being and the nurse's conscience. Do not assume that someone else on the treatment team or in the facility has taken or will take responsibility for treating the client within legal limits. The nurse's role as client advocate is especially important here. Commitment of a client to a treatment facility, the use of physical restraints, the use of medication or electroconvulsive therapy against the client's will must all be scrutinized and handled carefully by the nurse.

In any situation that might have legal ramifications, the nurse must know the law, must acutely observe, and must document those observations accurately. Good charting is essential and should be specific in all respects. For example, if a client is physically restrained, the nurse must chart the precipitating factors, situation, activities, and reason for restraints, the time and way in which the client was restrained, actions taken to meet the client's basic needs and rights (e.g., removing one limb restraint at a time and performing range of motion exercises, offering liquids, food, and commode), frequent, individual observations of the client for the duration of restraint, time the client was released from restraints, the client's behavior on release, and any other pertinent information.

Difficult situations may arise when the nurse and another member of the treatment team (e.g., a physician) disagree regarding the treatment of a client when legal considerations may be a factor. For example, the nurse may feel that a client is actively suicidal, while the other members of the treatment team feel that the client is ready for a weekend at home. In this kind of situation, the nurse must document all observations that led to this judgment and should seek help from the head nurse, nursing supervisor, director of nursing, or other administrators at the facility.

Clients with Legal Problems

Another potentially difficult situation is the treatment of a client who has been charged with or convicted of a violent crime, such as rape, domestic abuse, child abuse or molestation, incest, murder, or arson. Again, it is essential to be aware of legal factors pertinent to the client's treatment. For example, why is the client at the treatment facility? Has the court ordered observation to establish competence or insanity? Is treatment at this facility ordered by the court instead of or as part of sentence? Was the client being treated at the facility for another problem and during treatment confessed a crime to the staff?

If a client is at the facility for observation, it must be determined if there will indeed be any treatment involved, or if the staff will only observe the client. This observation, in any case, must then be accurate and well documented in the client's chart (a client's chart is a legal document and may be presented as evidence in court).

Examination of your own feelings about the client is crucial. The nurse must become and remain aware of his or her feelings in order to work effectively with the client and to remain nonjudgmental. For instance, whether you feel that the client "could not be guilty" or is "despicable . . . how could anyone do that sort of thing?" you will not be treating the client objectively. And yet it is realistic to expect that anyone working with the client will indeed have feelings about such a crime. Use staff conferences and interactions to ventilate and explore emotions and try to remain nonjudgmental toward the client.

The Aging Client

Aging is another difficult subject for many people, and often our discomfort influences our care of the older client. Respect for the individual and awareness of the feelings of both staff and client must work together to provide good nursing care that maintains the client's dignity. The aging client is a whole person with individual strengths and needs. Do not assume that a client over a certain age has organic brain syndrome, no longer has sexual feelings, or has no need for independence. It is important to promote independence to the client's optimum level of functioning no matter what the client's age. Provide the necessary physical care and assistance without drawing undue attention to the client's needs. Remember, the client may have never needed someone to care for him or her before and may feel humiliated by being in such a dependent position. The client may have previously been proud of his or her independence and have gained much self-esteem from this. This client may be horrified at the thought of "being a burden" and may experience despair. Do not dismiss the client's feelings as inappropriate due to your own discomfort; instead, encourage the client to express these feelings and give the client support while promoting as much independence for the client as possible. (See Care Plan 11, Grief Reaction.)

CARE PLANS

II

The *Manual of Psychiatric Nursing Care Plans* is intended as a resource in planning for each client's care. Because each client is an individual, with a unique background, home environment, support system, and particular set of behaviors, problems, strengths, needs, and goals, each client needs an individual plan of nursing care. The following care plans present information, behaviors or problems which a client may exhibit, possible short- and long-term goals, nursing objectives, and nursing actions for that problem or behavior complex. Because of individual differences and because the care plans in this manual are based on behaviors (as opposed to diagnoses or symptom complexes), plans should not be copied verbatim; some care plans in fact contain seemingly contradictory problems which call for different approaches. Therefore, each plan may be viewed as a resource from which to glean appropriate information and suggestions for use in each client's case. This manual focuses primarily on the client's behavior. We feel that this is essential, due to the uniqueness of each client, as well as to the fact that clients do not always present a textbook picture of a diagnosis or problem. Thus, this approach enables the nurse to use the manual in planning care in the absence of a specified psychiatric diagnosis. This is important since not all clients with emotional problems are found in psychiatric settings, diagnoses are not always immediately determined, and most important, good nursing care must involve seeing the client holistically rather than just in terms of a psychiatric diagnosis.

The nursing care process involves assessment; problem identification; determination of goals; identification of possible actions that would lead to resolutions; establishing deadlines or a timetable for evaluation; and revision of each step. Each part of this dynamic and continuing process is specific to the individual and must be determined for each client. The sections included in this manual are those which the authors found could be used as resources. In planning nursing care for each client, the nurse must supply timing, evaluation, and revision specific to the situation. The following is a brief explanation of each section to be found as a part of each care plan.

The section at the beginning of each care plan contains information about the behaviors or problems which may be helpful to know or recall when planning care for a client. The information included here may be of a background nature (e.g., types of psychoses in Care Plan 4, Chemical, Toxic, Physical Damage, or Intensive Care Unit Psychosis), include pertinent reminders (e.g., high-risk suicide factors in Care Plan 10, Suicidal Behavior), or may suggest other problems clients may experience (e.g., legal problems in Care Plan 26, Dependency or Inadequacy).

Behaviors or Problems. A range of behaviors and problems that the nurse may assess is listed in this section. Not all of the behaviors presented will be observed with each client, nor will all the problems necessarily be identified. Some behaviors may in fact appear contradictory. For example, sleep disturbances are usually noted in depressed clients. The Depression care plan notes both that the client may be unable to sleep or may sleep excessively. At the initial assessment, then, the nurse will identify the appropriate problem and proceed with the remainder of the care plan. Also, this section can help the nurse become aware of more of the client's potential problems since it lists possible problems, which may occur in concert with others.

Short- and Long-Term Goals. This section lists possible goals which the nurse (and the client) may identify to include in the client's care plan. These goals may be specific (e.g., Prevent electrolyte imbalance) or general (e.g., Build a trust relationship). The timing of implementing these goals should be made specific to individual clients, and the goals can then be evaluated and revised throughout the course of care.

Nursing Objectives and Nursing Actions. The objectives and approaches presented in this section are choices and alternatives that the nurse can select as means of achieving the short- and long-term goals. Specific practical suggestions are given, and often details are given for more than one approach so that care can be tailored to each individual. This section also includes important reminders in the implementation of care plans.

General Care Plans

The care plans in this section are intended to be used with each individual client's care plan because they address two of the most important facets of treatment: establishing the therapeutic relationship, and planning for the client's independence from treatment. In order for work with any client to be most effective, that work must be soundly based in a trusting relationship. The client and the nurse must see each other and their work as valuable, must strive toward mutually agreed-upon goals, and must enter into the problem-solving process together as described in Care Plan 1, Building a Trust Relationship.

Equally important is planning for the client's discharge from treatment or from the therapeutic relationship. Discharge planning should begin immediately when therapy begins, providing a focus for goals and an orientation toward as much independence as possible for the client. Discussing discharge plans with the client from the outset will help minimize the client's fears of discharge and will facilitate goal identification and an active role for the client in therapy. By using Care Plan 2, Discharge Planning, the nurse may anticipate the client's optimum level of functioning, the quality of the client's home situation and relationships with significant others, and the need for client-teaching throughout nursing care planning and implementation.

Building a Trust Relationship

The relationship a nurse has with a client can be viewed in four phases or stages:

1. *Introductory or orientation phase.* The purpose of the relationship is established and the roles of both the client and the nurse are defined.
2. *Testing phase.* During this time the client may become manipulative in an attempt to discover the limits of the relationship or test the nurse's sincerity and dependability. The client's attitude and behavior may vary a great deal, from pleasant and eager to please, to uncooperative or angry. This phase can be extremely trying and frustrating for the nursing staff.
3. *Working phase.* This is usually the longest phase of a trust relationship and the most overtly productive. The client begins to trust the staff, and begins to focus on problems or behaviors that need to be changed. During times of frustration the client may revert to testing behaviors. The staff should anticipate this and avoid becoming discouraged or giving up on the relationship.
4. *Termination phase.* Planning for terminating the relationship actually begins during the orientation phase of the relationship. As the client begins to rely more on herself or himself, plans for return to home or community, or a more permanent placement can be made. (See Care Plan 2, Discharge Planning.)

BEHAVIORS OR PROBLEMS

Difficulty trusting self

Difficulty trusting others, including authority figures

History of unsatisfactory relationships

Feelings of anxiety, fear, hostility, sadness, guilt, or inadequacy

Difficulties in relationships with significant others

Difficulties with others in school or work environment

Client's behavior may range from slightly withdrawn and quiet to openly hostile and aggressive, depending on the nature of the client's problems. (See other care plans as appropriate.)

SHORT-TERM GOALS

Develop a working relationship based on trust.

Establish the roles and responsibilities of the client and staff member within the therapeutic relationship.

Identify the behaviors or problems that led to the client's hospitalization.

LONG-TERM GOALS

Resolve the problems or behaviors that led to hospitalization.

Successfully terminate the client-staff relationship, resulting in the client's independence from the staff and hospital.

NURSING OBJECTIVES	NURSING ACTIONS
Introductory or Orientation Phase Define the purpose of the therapeutic relationship.	Introduce yourself to the client.
Establish the client's role and responsibilities.	Explain your role on the unit and within the milieu or treatment team.
Establish your (staff member's) role and responsibilities.	Obtain the client's perception of his or her problems and what the client expects to gain from the relationship or hospitalization.
	Assess the client's behavior, attitudes, problems, and needs.
	Make your expectations for the relationship clear to the client.
	Be honest in all interactions with the client. Avoid "glossing over" any unpleasant topics or circumstances. Take a matter-of-fact approach to such problems as commitment, legal involvement, and so forth.
Begin planning for termination of the relationship.	Let the client know you will work with her or him for a specified period of time, and that when the client is no longer in treatment, the relationship will end.
Testing Phase Set and maintain acceptable limits of the therapeutic relationship.	Be consistent with the client at all times.
	Show the client you accept him or her as a person. It is possible to accept the client, yet not accept "negative" behaviors.
	Avoid becoming the "only one" the client can talk to about his or her feelings and problems. This can be flattering, but is manipulative on the part of the client.
	Let the client know that pertinent information will be communicated to other staff members. Do not promise to keep information confidential as a way of obtaining the information.
	Set and maintain limits on the client's "negative" or unacceptable behavior; withdraw your attention from the client if necessary.
	Do not allow the client to bargain to obtain special favors or avoid following expectations to gain privileges.

NURSING OBJECTIVES (Continued)	NURSING ACTIONS (Continued)
	Give attention and positive feedback for acceptable or positive behavior.
	When limiting the client's behaviors, offer acceptable alternatives (e.g., "Don't throw ashtrays when you're angry—try punching your pillow instead.").
Working Phase Resolve the problems or behaviors that led to hospitalization.	Identify the behaviors and problems that led to hospitalization.
	Establish a regular schedule for meeting with the client (e.g., 1 hour each day, 10 minutes every hour), whatever fits your schedule and the client is able to tolerate.
	Inform the client how much time you have to spend at the beginning of the interaction.
	Tell the client when to expect you to return.
	Do whatever you say you will, and conversely, do not make promises you cannot keep. If extenuating circumstances prevent your following through, honestly explain this to the client. Expect and allow the client to be disappointed or angry; help him or her to express this appropriately and give support.
	Assist the client in identifying problem areas in her or his life situation.
	Encourage the client to ventilate feelings.
	Assist the client in identifying more effective methods of dealing with stress.
Termination Phase Terminate the relationship.	Assist the client in making plans for discharge (e.g., returning home, employment, etc.). (See Care Plan 2, Discharge Planning.)
	Anticipate the client's anxiety or insecurity about being discharged from the hospital and terminating the therapeutic relationship. The client may even revert to manipulative behavior or presenting problem behavior.
	Remember: The termination phase should actually begin in the introductory or orientation phase

	and should be reinforced as a goal and as a positive outcome throughout the entire therapeutic relationship.
Help the client establish an outside support system.	Assist the client in identifying sources of support outside the hospital, including agencies or individuals in community as well as significant others in his or her personal life.

It is important to obtain the following information:

Client's optimal level of functioning outside the hospital

Client's need for follow-up care, including frequency, type, location, or therapist

Client's ability to function independently before hospitalization

Type of situation to which the client is being discharged.

It may be necessary to consider:

Transfer to another hospital or institution

A sheltered setting

Other supportive services in the community

Relocation to a community other than the client's prehospitalization community.

Assess the client's motivations:

To stay in the hospital

To be discharged

To change out-of-hospital behavior or situation

To prevent readmission.

Remain aware of any secondary gains the client obtains from being hospitalized.

Remember: Discharge planning is a process that should begin on the client's admission to the hospital and should first be addressed in his or her initial care plan. Ideally, the client should work with the staff to develop an ongoing plan of care that is oriented to his or her discharge throughout the hospitalization.

BEHAVIORS OR PROBLEMS

Dependency on hospital

Dependency on hospital staff

Nonexistent or unrealistic goals and plans

Perception of discharge as a rejection by the staff and hospital system

Possible reappearance of original symptoms or the development of new symptoms

Lack of skills with which to function independently outside the hospital.

SHORT-TERM GOALS

Begin to terminate staff-client relationships.

Verbalize feelings about discharge.

Formulate concrete plans for the client's life situation:

1. Meeting essential physical needs (e.g., housing, employment, financial resources for adequate food, necessary transportation, and physical care if needed).
2. Meeting emotional needs through significant relationships, social activities, a general support system, and so forth.
3. Dealing with stress or problems.
4. Dealing with other facets of living specific to the client (e.g., legal problems, physical or health limitations, etc.).

LONG-TERM GOALS

Ability to meet essential needs (self-reliance when possible).

Eliminate any secondary gains from hospitalization.

Develop alternative ways to deal with stress or problems.

Identify community resources for crisis support.

Identify and contact resource persons in the community for various needs.

Terminate staff-client relationships.

NURSING OBJECTIVES	*NURSING ACTIONS*
Prepare the client for discharge, according to the disposition made by the treatment team (including the client, when possible).	On admission, ask the client about his or her expectations for hospitalization and plans for discharge. Attempt to keep the discharge plans as a focus for discussion throughout the client's hospitalization.
	Encourage the client to identify his or her goals and expectations after discharge.
	Help the client assess personal needs for specificity and structure. If it is indicated, assist the client in making a time schedule or other structure for activities (e.g., work, study, recreation, solitude, social activities, and significant relationships).
	Encourage the client to continue working toward goals that have been identified, but not yet realized during hospitalization (e.g., obtaining a high school diploma, vocational plans, divorce). Give positive support for goal identification and work begun.
Encourage the client to continue taking medications (if indicated) and continue with other therapy (e.g., outpatient visits, group therapy, relaxation techniques).	Talk with the client regarding medication or other treatment schedules and reasons for continuing therapy. Attempt to involve the client in treatment decisions to increase motivation and responsibility for follow-through with therapy on his or her own.
Prepare the client for future stresses, problems, etc.	Help the client identify factors in his or her life that have contributed to hospitalization (e.g., living situation, relationships, drug or alcohol use/abuse, work problems, inadequate coping mechanisms). Discuss each contributing factor, how the client sees these now, what can be changed, what the client is motivated to change, how the client will deal differently with these things to prevent rehospitalization.
Terminate the client-staff relationship without appearing to reject the client; minimize client's perception of rejection.	Always orient discussions with the client toward his or her eventual discharge.
Help the client deal with fears of discharge and reluctance to be discharged.	Support the client and give positive feedback when the client plans for discharge or talks positively about discharge.
Promote the client's self-confidence and independence.	Encourage the client to view discharge as a positive step or sign of growth, not as being "kicked out" of the hospital. Try to show this in your attitude toward the client.

Encourage the client to express feelings about leaving the hospital. Utilize groups, formal and informal, for clients to share feelings, discuss anticipated problems, fears, and ways to deal with the "outside world." (A "discharge group" that includes all clients who are near discharge may be helpful. It may also include a discussion of medications, their side effects, "when to call a physician," etc.)

Talk with the client about ways to meet personal needs after discharge (e.g., obtaining food, money, shelter, clothing, transportation, and a job).

Assess the client's skills and ability to meet the above needs (e.g., using phone and phone book, handling bank accounts and checkbook, contacting other community resources, setting up job interviews). Work with the client and obtain help from other disciplines if indicated (e.g., vocational rehabilitation, therapeutic education) to help the client develop the necessary skills before discharge.

Before discharge, encourage the client to make arrangements and other preparations as independently as possible (e.g., find housing, obtain a job, open bank accounts). Give support for doing this.

Through role-playing and setting up imaginary situations ("What will you do if . . . ?"), help the client anticipate problems and reinforce the client's problem-solving process.

Talk with the client about the feelings the client may experience after discharge (e.g., loneliness), and how the client will deal with these feelings.

Have occupational or recreational therapy services talk with the client about the use of leisure time, including hobbies, recreation, and exercise.

Do any indicated health teaching about medications, toxic symptoms and side effects, nutrition and exercise, and conditions such as diabetes or hypertension.

NURSING OBJECTIVES *(Continued)*	NURSING ACTIONS *(Continued)*
	Give the client a telephone number and name (if possible) to call in case of emergency.
	Do deliberately terminate your relationship with the client and talk with the client about this. First, try to acknowledge and deal with your own feelings about the client and the client's discharge; try not to merely withdraw attention from or avoid the client because he or she will be leaving. *Do not* encourage the client's further dependence on the staff members or hospital by encouraging the client to pay casual visits to the unit or by giving the client the home addresses or telephone numbers of staff members. It may be necessary to establish a policy that clients may not visit the unit after being discharged.
	Remember: It is generally not desirable for clients to become friends with staff members or to maintain social relationships after discharge.
Prepare client for transfer to another facility.	Give the client positive feedback regarding his or her progress, and discuss the need for further treatment.
	Point out the reasons for the transfer, if possible, such as need for long-term care, another type of care, different treatment structure, or another location. Involve the client in the decision-making process as much as possible and offer the client choices if possible.
	Stress that the transfer is not "punishment" (see "Termination of the client-staff relationship" above).
	Attempt to give the client information about his or her new environment; arrange a visit prior to the transfer, or provide the name of a contact person at the new facility.
Help client prepare for other aspects of discharge.	Work with other services as appropriate to meet the client's particular needs (e.g., day care, outpatient follow-up, vocational rehabilitation, or other community services).

Care Plans Related to Psychotic Behavior

Psychotic behavior may be encountered in clients who are experiencing a variety of problems and disorders. The care plans in this section address common types of psychotic symptoms (such as delusions and hallucinations) as well as problems or disorders which may produce psychotic behavior (such as schizophrenia, organic brain syndrome, or chemical, toxic, physical damage or ICU psychoses).

Psychotic behavior can include many different symptoms, resulting from disturbed throught processes, distorted perceptions, brain damage (either trauma-induced or from another physical cause), or chemical toxicity (due to alcohol or drug use, poison, or excessive levels of medications). The role of the nurse in working with a client who is exhibiting psychotic behavior may include providing nursing care in cooperation with other health care team members to treat the client's underlying problem, providing reality orientation, preventing injury to the client or others, helping the client build self-esteem and express feelings, or any number of other nursing interventions. All of the possible appropriate interventions may not be included in this section, but may be found in the care plans in the other sections of this manual.

Schizophrenia

Schizophrenia is a group of disorders manifested by characteristic disturbances of mood and behavior. The major types are:

Simple. Characterized by a slow, insidious loss of drive, ambition, and interests leading to a deterioration of mental processes and interpersonal relationships, and adjustment at a lower level of functioning.

Hebephrenic. Characterized by disorganized thinking, a shallow and inappropriate affect, giggling, silly, regressive behavior and mannerisms; frequently involves hypochondriacal complaints.

Catatonic. (1) Excited—characterized by excessive and sometimes violent motor activity and excitement; (2) Withdrawn—characterized by a generalized inhibition manifested by stupor, mutism, negativism, or waxy flexibility.

Schizo-affective. Characterized by a mixture of schizophrenic symptoms and pronounced elation or depression.

Paranoid. Characterized by persecutory or grandiose delusions, hallucinations, sometimes excessive religiosity, or hostile and aggressive behavior.

Chronic, undifferentiated. Mixed schizophrenic symptoms (of other types) are shown, along with disturbances of thought, affect, and behavior.

The prognosis is better (1) when the client has a history of good social, occupational, and sexual adjustment, (2) when the onset of the illness is acute, or (3) if a precipitating event was present.

Note also that the client will probably be taking medications such as major tranquilizers or antipsychotic agents.

BEHAVIORS OR PROBLEMS

Bizarre behavior
Withdrawn behavior
Regressive behavior
Increased anxiety, agitation
Low self-esteem
Loss of ego boundaries—an inability to perceive or differentiate the self from the external environment
Hallucinations
Delusions
Disorganized, illogical thinking
Inappropriate, inadequate emotional responses
Disturbance of self-initiated, goal-directed activity
Poor interpersonal relationships
Difficulty with verbal communication
Exaggerated responses to stimuli
Aggression toward self, others, or property
Sleep disturbances, fatigue
Appetite disturbances, inadequate nutrition
Sexual conflicts
Constipation
Menstrual disturbances

SHORT-TERM GOALS

Maintain adequate nutrition, elimination, rest, and activity.
Maintain a safe environment.
Establish rapport and build trust.
Assist the client to become a participant in the therapeutic community.
Increase the client's ability to communicate with others.
Decrease hallucinations, delusions, and other psychotic symptoms.

Reduce aggression or acting-out.
Increase self-esteem.

LONG-TERM GOALS

Identify and utilize strengths and assets, and develop a better self-image.

Reach and maintain maximal level of functioning.

Accept and deal effectively with the illness—its long-term nature, the need to remain on medications, and so forth as appropriate.

NURSING OBJECTIVES	*NURSING ACTIONS*
Decrease withdrawn behavior; provide goal-directed structured activity.	Spend time with the client even when he or she is unable to respond verbally or in a coherent manner. Convey your interest and caring.
	Make only those promises that you can realistically keep.
	Provide an opportunity for the client to learn that his or her feelings are valid and not so different from those of others.
	Limit the client's environment to enhance his or her feelings of security.
	Assign the same staff members to work with the client.
	Begin with one-to-one interactions, then progress to small groups as tolerated (introduce slowly).
	Establish and maintain a daily routine; explain any variation in this routine to the client.
Increase the client's self-esteem and feelings of self-worth.	Provide attention in a sincere, interested manner.
	Support any successes—ward responsibilities fulfilled, projects, interactions with staff members and other clients, etc.
	Help the client improve his or her grooming; assist when necessary in bathing, dressing, doing laundry, and so forth.
	Help the client accept as much responsibility for personal grooming as he or she can (don't do something for the client that he or she can do for self).
	Spend time with the client.
Orient the client to reality.	Reorient the client to person, place, and time as indicated (call the client by name, tell the client

NURSING OBJECTIVES (Continued)	NURSING ACTIONS (Continued)
	your name, tell the client where he or she is, the date, etc.).
Increase the client's ability to differentiate between the self and the external environment.	Help the client to establish what is real and unreal. Validate the client's real perceptions and correct the client's misperceptions in a matter-of-fact manner. Do not argue with the client, but do not give support for misperceptions.
Help the client reestablish ego boundaries.	Stay with the client if he or she is frightened; touching the client can sometimes be therapeutic. Evaluate the effectiveness of the use of touch on the individual client before using it consistently.
	Be simple, direct, and concise when speaking to the client.
	Talk with the client about simple, concrete things; avoid ideological or theoretical discussions.
	Direct activities toward helping the client accept and remain in contact with reality; use recreational or occupational therapy when appropriate.
Ensure a safe environment for the client.	Reassure the client that the environment is safe by explaining ward procedures, routines, tests, and so forth briefly and simply.
	Protect the client from self-destructive tendencies (remove items that could be used in self-destructive behavior).
	Be aware that the client may be considering actions that are harmful to self or others in response to auditory hallucinations.
Maintain a safe, therapeutic environment for other clients.	Remove the client from the group if his or her behavior becomes too bizarre, disturbing, or dangerous to others.
	Assist the client group to accept the client's "strange" behavior: give simple explanations to the client group as needed (e.g., "[client] is very sick right now; he needs our understanding and support").

	Consider other clients' needs and plan for at least one staff member to be available to other clients if several staff members are needed to care for this client.
Help the client work through regressive behavior.	*Remember:* Regression is a purposeful (conscious or unconscious) return to a lower level of functioning—an attempt to remove anxiety and reestablish equilibrium.
	Assess the client's present level of functioning and work from there.
	Make contact on the client's level of behavior, then help motivate him or her to bring regressed behavior in alignment with adult behavior. Assist the client to identify the unmet needs or feelings producing the regressive behavior. Encourage the client to express these feelings to help alleviate anxiety.
	Set realistic goals. Set daily goals and expectations.
	Make the client aware of your expectations of him or her.
	At first, do not offer choices to the client ("Would you like to go to activities?" "What would you like to eat?"); instead, approach client in directive manner ("It is time to eat," "Pick up your fork").
	Gradually, as the client tolerates, provide opportunities for him or her to accept responsibility and make personal decisions.
Maintain adequate hydration, nutrition, and elimination.	Be alert to the client's physical needs.
	Observe the client's patterns of food and fluid intake; you may need to monitor and record intake and output and daily weight. (See Care Plan 15, Client Who Will Not Eat.)
	Monitor the client's elimination patterns. Constipation occurs frequently due to use of major tranquilizers; you may need to administer a laxative to the client to establish regularity.

| --- | --- |
Decrease bizarre behavior, anxiety, agitation, or aggression.	Set limits on the client's behavior when he or she is unable to do so (when behavior interferes with other clients or becomes destructive). Do not use limit-setting to punish the client.
	Decrease excitatory stimuli in the environment; this client may not respond favorably to gym activities, competitive activities, or activities in large groups.
	Be aware of PRN medications and the client's varying need for them.
	See Care Plan 7, Hallucinations, Care Plan 6, Delusions, Care Plan 23, Hostility, and Care Plan 24, Aggressive Behavior.

Chemical, Toxic, Physical Damage, or Intensive Care Unit Psychosis

Psychosis caused by chemical, toxic, or physical damage, or sleep deprivation is usually acute, and will subside with treatment of the underlying cause. However, if the cause is irreversible, such as Korsakoff's syndrome, long-term treatment may be required. The major types of these psychoses are:

1. *Korsakoff's syndrome.* Results from chronic alcoholism and the associated vitamin B_1 (thiamine) deficiency. It usually occurs after a minimum of 5 to 10 years of heavy alcohol intake. The brain damage it causes is irreversible, even when further alcohol consumption is eliminated.

2. *Drug-induced psychosis.* Occurs most commonly following massive doses or chronic use of amphetamines; it clears in 1 to 2 weeks when drugs are discontinued. Also may result from use of hallucinogenic drugs (e.g., LSD); this lasts from 12 hours to 2 days. With repeated hallucinogen use, psychosis may occur briefly without recent drug ingestion. This psychosis usually occurs at ages 15 to 35.

3. *Endocrine imbalances.* Psychosis may result from intake of steroids, usually large doses resulting in toxic blood levels. Thyroid disturbances (*thyrotoxicosis*) produce psychotic behavior, which subsides spontaneously when thyroxin is brought to a therapeutic level.

4. *Sleep deprivation.* A client may experience psychosis with severe deprivation of rapid-eye-movement (REM) cycle sleep, usually associated with extreme stress. The most common example is "ICU psychosis." Clients in intensive care units experiencing constant stimuli (e.g., lights, sounds), disruption of diurnal patterns, interruption of sleep every 15 to 30 minutes, and so on, often exhibit psychotic behavior or symptoms.

BEHAVIORS OR PROBLEMS

Delusions (see Care Plan 6, Delusions)
Hallucinations (see Care Plan 7, Hallucinations)
Disorientation
Fear
Hostility
Physical acting-out (see Care Plan 24, Aggressive Behavior)
Disturbance of sleep patterns
Disturbance of eating habits (see Care Plan 15, Client Who Will Not Eat)
Inability to concentrate
Inattention to personal hygiene or grooming
Excessive environmental stimuli
Disrupted diurnal patterns
Impaired sleep cycle

SHORT-TERM GOALS

Prevent injury to the client and others.
Reorient to person, time, place, situation.
Maintain an adequate food and fluid intake.
Reassure the client's family or significant others when the psychotic behavior is related to temporary problems such as ICU psychosis. thyrotoxicosis, etc.
See Care Plan 3, Schizophrenia.

LONG-TERM GOALS

Adhere to medical treatment regime.
Avoid toxic substances to prevent recurrence.
Arrange for long-term treatment or placement if necessary.
Refer the client to the appropriate treatment facility if the psychotic behavior is related to alcohol or drug use or abuse.
See Care Plan 3, Schizophrenia.

NURSING OBJECTIVES	NURSING ACTIONS
Maintain adequate hydration, nutrition, and elimination.	Be alert to the client's physical needs.
	Observe the client's patterns of food and fluid intake; you may need to monitor and record intake and output and daily weight.
	Monitor the client's elimination patterns. Constipation occurs frequently due to use of major tranquilizers; you may need to administer a laxative to the client to maintain bowel regularity.
	See Care Plan 15, Client Who Will Not Eat.
Ensure a safe environment for the client.	Reassure the client that the environment is safe by explaining ward procedures, routine tests, and so forth, briefly and simply.
	Protect the client from self-destructive activities by removing items which could be used in self-destructive behavior.
	See Care Plan 10, Suicidal Behavior.
	Spend time with the client.
Orient the client to reality. Increase ability to differentiate between self and external environment. Help the client to reestablish ego boundaries.	Reorient the client to person, place, and time as necessary, by using the client's name often, telling the client your name, the date, the place, and so forth. Giving the client a calendar may be helpful.
	Evaluate the use of touch with the client. It may be reassuring and provide security for the client.
	Be simple, direct, and concise when speaking to the client.
	Talk with the client about simple, concrete things; avoid ideological or theoretical discussions.
	Direct activities toward helping the client accept and remain in contact with reality; use recreational or occupational therapy when appropriate.
Decrease bizarre behavior, anxiety, agitation, or aggression.	Set limits on the client's behavior when he or she is unable to do so (behavior that interferes with other clients or becomes self-destructive). Do not use limit-setting to punish the client.

Decrease excitatory stimuli in the environment; this client may not respond favorably to gym activities, competitive activities, or activities in large groups.

See Care Plan 7, Hallucinations, Care Plan 6, Delusions, Care Plan 23, Hostility, and Care Plan 24, Aggressive Behavior.

Organic Brain Syndrome

Organic brain syndrome may be gradual or acute in onset, depending on the etiology. It may be accompanied by psychosis (see Care Plan 4, Chemical, Toxic, Physical Damage, or ICU Psychosis); some clients may exhibit occasional, sporadic insight into behavior or have periods of lucidity. The amount of brain damage is not always proportional to the client's mental status. For example, a client with a small area of brain damage may have a high degree of dysfunction and vice versa. *Remember*: Organic brain syndrome is *not* always part of the aging process. Do not assume an elderly client will be forgetful, confused, etc.

Some major causes of organic brain syndrome are:

1. *Cerebral arteriosclerosis.* Results in diminished blood supply and oxygen to the cerebral cortex. Initial symptoms are simple forgetfulness, short attention span, and decreased ability to concentrate. Progression of the disease may result in psychosis. It usually occurs at ages 60 to 70.
2. *Senile dementia.* Results from diffuse, primary degeneration and loss of brain neurons. Cerebral atrophy, especially of the frontal lobes, occurs. The client's behavior becomes uninhibited, socially inappropriate, or embarrassing. It usually occurs at ages 70 to 80.
3. *Posttrauma.* Results from brain damage following trauma to the cerebrum. The cerebral injury may be due to hemorrhage, a direct blow, laceration, etc. This can occur at any age.

BEHAVIORS OR PROBLEMS

Confusion
Disorientation
Short attention span
Inability to concentrate
Impaired performance of daily living activities (e.g., grooming and personal hygiene)
Inappropriate social behavior (e.g., use of profanity or sexual behaviors inappropriate to the place or situation)
Fear
Feelings of hopelessness
Inability to deal with abstract thoughts or ideas
Withdrawn behavior
Impaired memory, particularly of recent events
Lack of reasonable judgment
Disturbance of sleep patterns (the client may wander or become more confused at night)
Disinterest in surroundings
Delusions (see Care Plan 6, Delusions)
Hallucinations (see Care Plan 7, Hallucinations)
Combative behavior (see Care Plan 23, Hostility and Care Plan 24, Aggressive Behavior)
Inadequate food and fluid intake (see Care Plan 15, Client Who Will Not Eat)

SHORT-TERM GOALS

Maintain adequate nutritional and fluid intake.
Prevent electrolyte imbalance.
Protect the client from injury.
Orient the client to reality.
Decrease hallucinations and delusions.

LONG-TERM GOALS

Reach his or her optimal level of independence.
Form satisfactory social relationships within his or her own limitations.
Live in as nonrestrictive environment as possible. (See Care Plan 2, Discharge Planning.)
Exhibit appropriate social behavior.

NURSING OBJECTIVES	NURSING ACTIONS
Maintain adequate food and fluid intake. Prevent electrolyte imbalance. Maintain adequate elimination.	Offer the client small amounts of food frequently, including juices, liquids, malts and fortified liquids. Monitor the client's bowel movements; do not allow impaction to occur. *Remember*: The client's inactivity, ingestion of any major tranquilizers, and decreased food intake can cause constipation. Provide a quiet environment with decreased stimuli at mealtimes. Feed the client if necessary. (See Care Plan 15, Client Who Will Not Eat.)
Provide a safe environment. Prevent injury to the client and to others.	Assess the client's ability to ambulate independently if he or she is elderly or physically disabled; assist the client until you are sure of physical independence. Observe the client or know his or her whereabouts at all times. Check the client frequently at night. *Remember*: Confusion or disorientation may increase at night. Provide adequate light in the environment, especially at night. Provide adequate restraints (e.g., Posey, vest, etc.) if necessary for protection. *Note*: Side rails alone may prove dangerous if the client tries to climb over them.
Facilitate adequate rest and sleep.	Provide activity and stimulation during the day. Do not allow the client to sleep all day or he or she will be awake at night. Provide a regular nightly routine, such as a tepid bath, and a quiet environment. Utilize bedtime medication for sleep if necessary. *Remember*: Sedatives or hypnotics can increase restlessness and confusion in the elderly; closely observe the client for their effects. Also, the dosage may need to be decreased for the elderly.

NURSING OBJECTIVES (Continued)	NURSING ACTIONS (Continued)
Orient the client to reality. Decrease confusion. Facilitate memory. Increase interest in the environment.	Assess the client's disorientation or confusion regularly. Refer to the date, time of day, and recent activities during your interactions with the client. Correct errors in the client's perception of reality in a matter-of-fact manner. Do not laugh at the client's misperceptions, and do not allow other clients to ridicule the client. Encourage visits from the client's friends and family and assess their effect on the client's confusion and memory. You may need to limit the visits if the client tolerates them poorly. Allow the client to have familiar personal possessions in his or her room—pictures and own clothing are usually helpful. Assign the same staff members to work with the client whenever possible to decrease his or her confusion. Initially, it is easier for the client to relate to a few familiar people.
Decrease delusions or hallucinations.	See Care Plan 6, Delusions and Care Plan 7, Hallucinations.
Facilitate adequate grooming, hygiene, and other activities of daily living.	Explain any task to be done in short simple steps. Instruct the client, using clear direct sentences, to do one part of the task at a time. Tell the client your expectations directly. Do not ask the client to choose unnecessarily (e.g., tell the client it is time to eat rather than asking the client if he or she wants to eat). Allow the client an ample amount of time to perform any given task; it may take the client much longer to dress or comb hair because of a lack of concentration and a short attention span. Remain patient throughout the task; do not attempt to "hurry" the client. This will frustrate him or her and make the task completion impossible. Assist the client as needed to maintain daily functions and adequate personal hygiene.

NURSING OBJECTIVES (Continued)	NURSING ACTIONS (Continued)
	Do not confuse the client with reasons "why" things are to be done; abstract ideas will not be comprehended.
Decrease socially inappropriate behavior and facilitate the development of acceptable social skills.	Do not allow the client to embarrass himself or herself in front of others. Intervene as soon as you observe such behavior (e.g., undressing, advances toward others, urinating somewhere other than commode).
	Take a matter-of-fact approach: do not chastise or ridicule the client.
	Offer acceptable alternatives, and redirect the client's activities (e.g., "Mr. X, it is not appropriate to undress here, I'll help you to your room to undress.").
	Praise the client for appropriate behavior.
Increase interest in the surroundings.	Determine what the client's interests, hobbies, and favorite activities were before hospitalization. (It may be necessary to obtain information from the client's family or friends.)
Increase ability to concentrate.	Assess the client's current capability of engaging in former hobbies or activities, and make them available as much as possible.
Lengthen attention span.	
Decrease feelings of hopelessness.	Introduce the activities during a time of day when the client seems most able to concentrate and participate.
	Approach the client with a calm, positive attitude. Convey the idea that you believe he or she can succeed.
	Begin with small short-term activities to make successful completion easier.
	Increase the length or complexity of the task gradually.
	Assess the activities and approaches, determine those that are most successful, and continue to utilize them.
	Encourage interaction about an activity or small-group activities with clients sharing similar interests.

NURSING OBJECTIVES *(Continued)*	NURSING ACTIONS *(Continued)*
	Allow the client to ventilate feelings of despair or hopelessness. Do not merely try to "cheer up" the client or belittle his or her feelings by using pat phrases or platitudes.

Delusions

Delusions are fixed false beliefs which have no basis in reality. Clients may have several types of delusions. A client may have insight into the delusional state but may be unable to alter it. The client is attempting to meet some need through the delusion, such as an increased self-esteem, security, reassurance, punishment, freedom from anxiety associated with feelings of guilt, fear, and so forth. Clients (especially those with paranoia) may have *fixed delusions*—delusions that may persist throughout their lives. Many psychotic clients have *transient delusions*—delusions that do not persist over time. Three phases have been identified in this process of delusional thinking: first, the client is totally involved in delusions; second, reality testing and trust in others coexist with the delusions, and third, the client no longer experiences delusions. *Remember*: Delusions are a protection and can be abandoned only when the client feels adequate and secure. Delusions are not within the client's conscious control.

BEHAVIORS OR PROBLEMS

Delusions of control
Delusions of grandeur
Delusions of persecution
Delusions of infidelity (regarding self or partner)
Ideas of reference
Delusions of being accused
Delusions of wealth
Delusions of poverty
Delusions of contamination
Somatic delusions
Paranoid delusions
Delusions regarding eating and food

SHORT-TERM GOALS

Assist the client to feel safer and more secure in the environment.
Build self-esteem.
Integrate the client into the therapeutic community.
Encourage the client to trust staff members and others enough to confide his or her delusional thinking.

LONG-TERM GOALS

Regarding transient delusions:
Eliminate pathological delusions.
Resume responsibilities of life in the client's home community.
Regarding fixed delusions:
Increase recognition of delusions and the client's ability to cope with delusions.
Increase the client's ability to function in his or her home environment.

NURSING OBJECTIVES	NURSING ACTIONS
Help the client feel as secure and accepted as possible.	See Care Plan 1, Building a Trust Relationship.
Build a trust relationship.	Be sincere and honest in communicating with the client. Avoid vague or evasive remarks.
	Be consistent in setting forth expectations, enforcing rules, and so forth.
	Do not make promises that you cannot keep.
	Encourage the client to talk with you, but do not pry or cross-examine for information.
	Explain procedures before carrying them out (try to be sure the client understands the procedure).
Assist to increase the client's self-esteem.	Give positive feedback for the client's successes.
	Recognize and support the client's accomplishments (e.g., activities or projects completed, ward responsibilities fulfilled, or interactions initiated).
	Engage the client in one-to-one activities at first, then activities in small groups, and gradually activities in large groups.
Decrease the client's anxiety and fears; help the client feel at ease.	Recognize the client's delusions as the client's perception of the environment.
	Initially, do not argue with the client or try to convince the client that the delusions are false or unreal.
	Interact with the client on the basis of real things; do not dwell on the delusional material.
	Show empathy regarding the client's feelings; reassure the client of your presence and acceptance.
	Do not be judgmental or belittle or joke about the client's beliefs.
Help the client recognize delusions as such.	Never convey to the client that you accept the delusions as reality.

NURSING OBJECTIVES (Continued)	NURSING ACTIONS (Continued)
	Directly interject doubt regarding delusions as soon as the client seems ready to accept this. Do not argue with the client, but do present a factual account of the situation as you see it.
	Attempt to discuss the delusional thoughts as a problem in the client's life; can the client see that the delusions interfere with his or her life?
Assist the client in finding healthy ways of dealing with feelings of anxiety, fear, and low self-esteem, independent of delusions.	Encourage the client to ventilate feelings; support his or her attempts to verbalize anxiety, fears, and so forth, directly.
	Explore with the client various ways to express and deal with feelings; help the client identify ways that are effective and acceptable.
Decrease or eliminate delusions regarding food and eating: —that others are deprived of food if client eats;	Seat the client with a group of clients who also are eating.
	The client may eat if the food is placed where no staff member can observe the client's eating.
	It may help to spoon-feed the client.
—that food is contaminated;	Using disposable plates, cups, and utensils may be helpful.
	Food may be brought for the client from his or her home.
	It may help if the staff members eat with the client.
	Serve the client foods in containers that can be opened by the client (e.g., milk cartons).
	Serve food in skins or shells (like potatoes, eggs, oranges, bananas, or grapefruit) and allow the client to view their preparation or allow the client to prepare.
—that the food is poisoned.	Gaining the client's trust is extremely important (see Care Plan 1, Building a Trust Relationship).
	Let other clients (or staff) be served and begin eating before the client so that the client can see them eat.

NURSING OBJECTIVES (Continued)	NURSING ACTIONS (Continued)
	It may be helpful if the client helps to serve the food.
	Let the client select his or her own food from the cafeteria.
	Always suggest verbally and nonverbally, that client will find eating pleasurable.
	Note: Some of the above measures may be helpful in terms of increasing the client's nutritional intake, but they must be done without validating the client's delusional system. They must be done unobtrusively and should be employed initially if the client's nutritional status is severely impaired. As a trust relationship develops, gradually introduce other foods and more routine procedures.
	See also Care Plan 15, Client Who Will Not Eat.

Hallucinations

Hallucinations are perceptions of an external stimulus without a source in the external world. They may involve any of the senses—sight, sound, smell, touch, taste. Clients often act on these inner perceptions, which may become more compelling to them than external reality. Hallucinations may occur with any of the following conditions (see other care plans as appropriate):

Withdrawal from alcohol, barbiturates, meprobamate, other substances
Generalized organic brain disease
Schizophrenia
Hallucinogenic drugs (e.g., mescaline, LSD, PCP)
Drug toxicity (e.g., amphetamine psychosis, digitalis toxicity)
Manic-depressive psychosis, severe mania
Alcoholic hallucinosis (the client may be oriented to person, place, and time while hallucinating)
Endocrine imbalance (e.g., steroid psychosis, thyrotoxicosis)
Sleep or sensory deprivation

Remember: The hallucination seems very real to the client. The client may perceive the hallucination as reality rather than his or her actual external surroundings, or the client may be aware that he or she is hallucinating. The hallucination may be related to an inability to distinguish and discriminate among incoming stimuli (for example, noise from the next room may be perceived or distorted as more real or more immediate than a person's voice speaking directly to the client).

BEHAVIORS OR PROBLEMS

Hallucinations (auditory, visual, tactile, or olfactory)
Fear and insecurity
Agitation
Aggression toward self, others, or property (see Care Plan 24, Aggressive Behavior)
Inability to discriminate between real and unreal perceptions
Guilt, remorse, or embarrassment on realization of hallucinatory experiences
Manipulative behavior (e.g., avoiding activities or other responsibilities by reason of "hallucinations")
Delusions (see Care Plan 6, Delusions)
Refusal to eat (see Care Plan 15, Client Who Will Not Eat)

SHORT-TERM GOALS

Provide safety for the client and others.
Decrease stimuli in the client's environment.
Interrupt the pattern of hallucinations; replace them with real interactions and activities with other people.
Decrease the client's fear, anxiety, or agitation.

LONG-TERM GOALS

Establish satisfying relationships with people.
Establish patterns of working through fear, anxiety, and anger in a manner that the client feels is safe and acceptable, independent of hallucinations or other psychotic symptoms.
Understand the hallucinatory process.
Plan for the possible recurrence of hallucinations.

NURSING OBJECTIVES	NURSING ACTIONS
Prevent the client from harming self, others, or property.	Provide protective supervision for the client, but avoid "hovering" over the client.
	Remain aware of cues indicating that the client is hallucinating (e.g., intent listening for no apparent reason, talking to "someone" when no one is present, muttering to self, inappropriate facial expression).
	See also Care Plan 23, Hostility, Care Plan 24, Aggressive Behavior, and Care Plan 10, Suicidal Behavior.
Interrupt the client's pattern of hallucinations.	Be aware of all surrounding stimuli, including sounds from other rooms (e.g., television or stereo in adjacent areas).
	Try to decrease stimuli or move the client to another area.
	Avoid conveying to the client the belief that hallucinations are real. Do *not* converse with the "voices," or otherwise reinforce the client's belief in the hallucination as reality.
	Communicate with the client verbally in direct, concrete, specific terms. Avoid gesturing, abstract ideas, and giving opportunity for choices.
Encourage the client's contact with real people, interactions, and activities.	Respond verbally to anything real that the client talks about; reinforce the client's conversation when he or she refers to present reality.
	Encourage the client to make staff members aware of hallucinations—when they occur or when they interfere with the client's ability to converse and carry out activities.
	If the client appears to be hallucinating, attempt to engage the client's attention and provide conversation or a concrete activity of interest to the client.
	Keep to simple, basic topics of conversation to provide a base in reality.
	Provide simple activities that can be easily or realistically accomplished by the client (e.g., crocheting or crafts projects).

NURSING OBJECTIVES (Continued)	NURSING ACTIONS (Continued)
	If the client tolerates it, use touch in a non-threatening manner to provide a reality base; allow the client to touch your arm or hand.
Decrease the client's fear, anxiety, or agitation.	Provide a structured environment with as many routine activities of daily living as possible. Explain unexpected changes. Make your expectations clear to the client in simple, direct terms.
	Be alert for signs of increasing fear, anxiety, or agitation so you may intervene as early as possible and prevent harm to the client, others, or property.
	Intervene with one-to-one contact, seclusion, and PRN medication (as ordered) as appropriate.
	Avoid "backing the client into a corner" either physically or verbally.
	Be realistic in your expectations of the client: do not expect more (or less) of the client than the client is capable of.
	Build a trust relationship (see Care Plan 1, Building a Trust Relationship).
Help the client express fear, anxiety, or any other feelings he or she has.	Encourage the client to ventilate his or her feelings; first in one-to-one contacts, then in small groups, then in larger groups as tolerated.
	Help the client explore and identify ways to relieve anxiety when the client is able to verbalize such feelings.
Help relieve the client's guilt, remorse, or embarrassment when the client remembers his or her psychotic behavior.	Encourage ventilation of feelings; be supportive.
	Show acceptance of the client's behavior, and of the client as a person; do not joke about or judge the client's behavior.
Help the client anticipate ways to deal with a possible future recurrence of hallucinations.	See Care Plan 2, Discharge Planning.

Care Plans Related to Affect

Affect, or mood, can be described as an emotional tone, feeling, or reaction to experience. Disturbances in affect can be manifested by a wide range of behaviors, such as suicidal thoughts and behavior, withdrawn behavior, or a profound increase or decrease in the client's level of psychomotor activity. The care plans in this section address the behaviors and problems most directly related to affect, but the care plans in the other sections of the manual may also be appropriate in the planning of a particular client's care (for example, Care Plan 21, Withdrawn Behavior).

Problems related to affect may result from a psychiatric disorder (e.g., bipolar affective disorder or manic-depressive illness), a crisis or loss in a client's life (see Care Plan 11, Grief Reaction), or some other condition (such as depressive neurosis), situation, or problem. Regardless of the specific cause of the client's problem, however, encouraging and facilitating the expression of feelings is a nursing intervention commonly found in these care plans, since many times the client has great difficulty recognizing and ventilating his or her feelings. In this work, it is important that the nurse, too, acknowledge and work through personal feelings so that they do not interfere with the therapeutic nature of the client-nurse relationship.

Manic Behavior

Manic behavior, also called bipolar affective disorder, is characterized by a past history of "high" and "low" moods with periods of relatively normal and effective functioning in between. The onset of the illness is usually between ages 20 and 40. Studies indicate that there is a strong hereditary component to the illness. Parents of the client frequently have a history of alcoholism. The client frequently abuses alcohol, sometimes in an attempt to self-medicate, or the client may have both problems—bipolar affective disorder and alcoholism—each of which necessitates treatment.

Lithium carbonate is frequently the drug of choice. This drug may be contraindicated in clients with impaired liver, renal, or cardiac function. Monitoring of the serum lithium level at specified intervals is required. See the Nursing Objectives and Nursing Actions sections below for a listing of signs and symptoms that may indicate toxic or near-toxic blood levels.

BEHAVIORS OR PROBLEMS

Hyperactivity, increased agitation
Grandiose schemes and plans
Loose associations (loosely and poorly associated ideas)
Push of speech (rapid, forced speech)
Tangentiality of ideas and speech
Decreased concentration, short attention span
Inappropriate, bizarre, flamboyant dress or use of make-up
Buying sprees
Insomnia
Fatigue
Poor nutritional and fluid intake
Hostile behavior (see Care Plan 23, Hostility, Care Plan 25, Passive-Aggressive or Manipulative Behavior)
Threatened aggression toward self and others (see Care Plan 24, Aggressive Behavior and Care Plan 10, Suicidal Behavior)
Hallucinations (see Care Plan 7, Hallucinations)
Delusions (see Care Plan 6, Delusions)
Sexual acting out; flirtatious, seductive behavior

SHORT-TERM GOALS

Decrease hyperactivity, agitation, hallucinations, etc.
Establish and maintain adequate biological functioning in the areas of nutrition, hydration, elimination, rest, and sleep.

LONG-TERM GOALS

Educate the client and his or her family to understand the illness, its genetic component, the use of chemotherapy, and the signs and symptoms of toxicity.
Accept the need for continuing chemotherapy and for frequent blood tests as indicated by the physician.

NURSING OBJECTIVES	NURSING ACTIONS
Establish rapport and build trust relationship.	Show acceptance of the client as a person.
	Use firm, yet calm, relaxed approach.
	Avoid making promises you cannot realistically keep.
	Assign the client to the same staff members when possible (keep in mind the staff member's ability to work with a manic client for extended periods of time).
Decrease hyperactivity, anxiety, and agitation.	Decrease environmental stimuli whenever possible.
	Respond to cues of increased restlessness or agitation by removing stimuli and perhaps isolating the client; a private or single occupancy room may be beneficial.
	Limit group activities until the client can tolerate that level of stimuli.
	Administer chemotherapy (probably will be lithium carbonate or phenothiazines initially). Use PRN medication judiciously, preferably before the client's behavior becomes out of control.
	Provide a consistent, structured environment. Let the client know what is expected of him or her. Set goals with the client as soon as it becomes possible to do so.
	Give simple, direct explanations for routine actions, procedures, tests, and so forth. Do not argue with the client.
	Encourage the client to verbalize his or her feelings of anxiety, anger, or fear. Explore ways to relieve stress and tension with the client as soon as it is possible to do so.
Provide physical activity or outlet for relief of tension and energy.	Help the client plan activities within his or her scope of achievement. Remember that the client's attention span is short and plan accordingly.
	Avoid highly competitive activities.

NURSING OBJECTIVES (Continued)	NURSING ACTIONS (Continued)
	Evaluate how much stimuli and responsibility the client can tolerate with respect to group activities, interactions with others, or visitors and attempt to limit these accordingly.
Promote rest and sleep.	Provide time for a rest period, nap, or quiet time during the client's daily schedule.
	Observe the client closely for signs of fatigue. Monitor his or her sleep patterns.
	Decrease stimuli before the client retires (e.g., dim lights, turn down television, provide a warm bath).
	Utilize comfort measures or sleeping medication if needed.
	Encourage the client to follow a routine of sleeping at night (limit interaction with the client at night) rather than during the day (allow only a short nap during the day).
Encourage a nutritious diet.	Monitor the client's eating patterns, food and fluid intake. You may need to record intake and output, calorie count, and protein intake.
	The client may need a high-protein, high-calorie diet with supplemental feedings.
	Provide foods that the client can carry with him or her if unable to sit and eat (e.g., milkshakes, sandwiches, "finger foods").
	See Care Plan 15, Client Who Will Not Eat.
Assist the client in meeting his or her basic needs and in carrying out necessary activities of daily living.	Monitor the client's elimination pattern (constipation is frequently a problem).
	Help the client to meet as many of his or her personal needs as possible.
	If help is needed, assist the client with personal hygiene, including mouthcare, bathing, dressing, and laundering clothes.
Provide emotional support.	Give the client positive feedback when appropriate.

NURSING OBJECTIVES *(Continued)*	NURSING ACTIONS *(Continued)*
	Structure tasks at which the client will succeed—short-term, simple projects or responsibilities, occupational or recreational therapy activities.
	Encourage the client's appropriate expression of feelings regarding future treatment plans or discharge plans. Support any realistic goals and plans the client proposes.
Provide the client and his or her family with education about lithium carbonate therapy.	Inform the client and his or her family about lithium carbonate: dosage, the need to take it only as prescribed, the toxic symptoms (see below), the need for blood tests (to monitor serum lithium level) as physician prescribes, salt and diet considerations (any condition which depletes salt in body—crash diets, increase in perspiration, vomiting or diarrhea—may increase serum lithium level).
Promote compliance with lithium carbonate therapy.	
	Explain in clear simple terms. Reinforce teaching with written material as indicated.
	Stress to the client and the client's family that lithium carbonate must be taken regularly and continually to be effective; that just because the client "feels better" or because his or her mood is level is *NOT* sufficient cause to discontinue the drug.
	The side effects that can be expected from lithium carbonate therapy include:*
	Mild intermittent nausea Thirst, increased liquid intake, increased urination Metallic taste Slight intermittent hand tremor.
	The signs that may indicate a near-toxic blood level of lithium carbonate, which the client should report to a health professional include:
	Insatiable thirst Persistent diarrhea Persistent vomiting Lack of coordination

*The lists of signs and symptoms are taken from *The Patient's Guide to Lithium*, by Kathryn R. Kucera-Bozarth. Copyright © 1979 by the Missouri Department of Mental Health. All rights reserved. Used by permission.

Muscular weakness
Dizziness
Blurred vision
Slurred speech
Trembling of the hands
Difficulty concentrating
Decreased speed of thinking
Confusion
Buzzing, ringing, or whistling in the ears.

The client should be encouraged to see a physician or to go to an emergency room immediately if these signs of toxicity occur:

No feeling in the skin
Movement of eyeballs side-to-side
Muscle twitching
Restlessness
Jerking or twisting of arms or legs
Loss of bladder or bowel control
"Blackout" episodes, convulsions or seizures
Stupor (may lead to coma).

Depression

Grief is the result of a "normal" depressive response to a loss (see Care Plan 11, Grief Reaction).

Reactive depression or depressive neurosis is manifested by an excessive reaction of depression due to internal conflict or to an identifiable event.

Involutional melancholia is the anxious, agitated, delusional depression of the menopausal years, lasting up to several months' duration. There is no known precipitating factor; concern centers around realization of the aging process and its effect on the client's life.

Psychotic depression is a depression so profound that the client loses contact with reality, develops delusions, and is frequently a suicide risk.

Manic-depressive illness, depressed type: apprehension, perplexity, uneasiness, and agitation are manifested. Hallucinations and delusions (usually of guilt or of hypochondriacal or paranoid ideas) may occur.

Depression is frequently seen in clients during alcohol or other drug withdrawal. Depressed behavior may also be seen in a number of other disorders or behaviors, such as anorexia nervosa, schizophrenia, and so forth. (See other care plans as appropriate.)

BEHAVIORS OR PROBLEMS

Sleep disturbances: early awakening, insomnia, or excessive sleeping

Disturbances of appetite and regular eating patterns, weight gain or loss (see Care Plan 15, Client Who Will Not Eat)

Constipation

Poor personal hygiene

Decreased motor activity

Slowed mental processes

Verbalization diminished in quantity, quality, and spontaneity

Low self-esteem

Overall lack of energy for purposeful activity

Fatigue

Generalized restlessness, agitation

Anxiety

Hallucinations (see Care Plan 7, Hallucinations)

Anger, hostility (usually not overt) (see Care Plan 23, Hostility)

Delusions (see Care Plan 6, Delusions)

Suicidal ideas or behavior (see Care Plan 10, Suicidal Behavior)

Grieving process (see Care Plan 11, Grief Reaction)

SHORT-TERM GOALS

Prevent the client from harming himself or herself.

Establish and maintain adequate biological functioning in the areas of nutrition, hydration, elimination, rest and sleep.

Establish and maintain adequate personal hygiene.

Express and ventilate feelings, both verbally and nonverbally.

Channel anger or hostility outward in a safe manner.

Orient the client to reality.

Develop or increase feelings of self-worth.

LONG-TERM GOALS

Accept loss (if any), and adapt lifestyle to that loss.

Resolve internal conflict.
Increase feelings of confidence and self-worth.
Increase ability to cope with anxiety and stress.
Reestablish and maintain relationships and a social life.
Assume the responsibility of dealing with feelings—find others to talk to and establish a support system.
Return to former community, occupation, and so forth, as appropriate and desired by client.
Make future plans (see Care Plan 2, Discharge Planning).

NURSING OBJECTIVES	*NURSING ACTIONS*
Maintain adequate nutrition, hydration, and elimination.	Closely observe the client's food and fluid intake. Record intake and output if necessary.
	Offer the client foods that are easily chewed, fortified liquids such as orange juice with nutritional supplement and high protein malts. If the client is overeating, limit access to foods, kitchen; schedule meals and snacks; serve limited portions. Give the client positive feedback for adhering to prescribed diet.
	Try to find out what foods the client likes and make them available at meals and for snacks.
	Do not tell the client he or she will get sick or die from not eating or drinking; this may be the client's wish. See Care Plan 15, Client Who Will Not Eat.
	Observe and record the client's pattern of bowel elimination. Depressed clients may become severely constipated as a result of the depression, inadequate exercise, inadequate food and fluid intake, or some medications.
	Encourage good fluid intake to prevent constipation.
	Be aware of PRN laxative orders and the possible need to offer medication to the client, as the client may not be aware of constipation or ask for medication.
Provide an adequate balance of rest, sleep, and activity.	If the client withdraws to his or her bed and sleeps excessively:
	—Client may need physical assistance to get up, dress, and spend time on the unit (if the client is ambulatory).
	—Be gentle but firm in setting limits regarding time spent in bed; set specific time when client

	must be up in the morning, when and how long client may rest.
	If the client cannot sleep:
	—Provide a quiet, peaceful time for resting.
	—Provide a nighttime routine or comfort measures (e.g., backrub, tepid bath, warm milk) to facilitate sleep.
	—Talk with the client only for brief period(s) during night hours to help relieve anxiety and to provide reassurance before the client returns to bed.
	—Do not allow the client to sleep for long periods during the day.
	—Use PRN medications as indicated to facilitate sleep. (*Note:* Some medications used for sleep may worsen depression or cause agitation in depressed persons.)
	—Decrease environmental stimuli (e.g., loud conversation, bright lights) in late evening.
	—Limit coffee (or other caffeine) consumption, especially in the evening or at night.
Prevent the client from harming self.	Provide a safe environment for the client.
	Continually assess the client's potential for suicide.
	Closely observe the client (it may be desirable to place the client in a bedroom near the nursing station), especially at these vulnerable times:
	—After antidepressant medication begins to raise mood.
	—After any sudden, dramatic behavioral change (e.g., sudden cheerfulness, relief, freedom from guilt, or giving away personal belongings).
	—Unstructured time on the unit.

	—Times when the number of staff is limited (e.g., change of shift report times, night shift).
	See Care Plan 10, Suicidal Behavior.
Build a trust relationship.	Initially, assign the same staff members to work with the client whenever possible.
	When approaching the client, use a moderate, level tone of voice. Avoid being overly cheerful.
	Use silence and active listening when interacting with the client. Let the client know you are concerned and that you consider the client a worthwhile person.
	Avoid asking the client many questions, especially questions which require only brief answers. Interact with the client on topics with which the client is comfortable. Do not probe for information.
	When first communicating with the client, use simple, direct sentences; avoid complex sentences or directions.
Develop or increase feelings of self-worth.	As necessary, assist the client to have good personal hygiene and appearance with baths, clean hair, clean clothes, haircut, etc., as appropriate.
	At first, provide simple activities, which can be easily and quickly accomplished. Begin with a project on the unit with the client alone; progress to group occupational and recreational therapy sessions.
	Give the client honest praise for the accomplishment of small activities, ward or individual responsibilities, realizing how difficult it can be for the client to perform these tasks.
	Gradually increase the amount and complexity of activities or responsibilities expected of the client; give positive feedback at each level of accomplishment.
	It may be necessary to stress to the client that he or she should begin *doing* things in order to *feel* better, rather than waiting to *feel* better before *doing* things.

| --- | --- |
Relieve depression.	Encourage the client to ventilate his or her feelings in whatever ways he or she is comfortable with—verbal and nonverbal. Let the client know you will listen and accept what he or she is expressing.
	Be comfortable sitting with the client in silence. Let the client know that you are available to talk, but don't require the client to converse. You can be nonverbally supportive with only your caring presence.
	Allow (and encourage) the client to cry. Stay with and support the client if he or she desires or provide privacy if the client wishes to be alone.
	Don't cut off interaction with cheerful remarks or platitudes (such as, "No one really wants to die," "Of course life is worth living," or "You'll feel better soon"). Do not belittle the client's feelings. Accept the client's verbalizations of feelings as real and give support for this ventilation of feelings, especially for expression of emotions that may be difficult for the client to accept in himself or herself (like anger).
	Assist the client in problem-solving and making changes in behavior, caring for self, and discharge planning. (See Care Plan 2, Discharge Planning.)

Suicidal Behavior

Suicide is one of the 10 leading causes of death in the United States and is increasing among people aged 15 to 24. Men commit suicide more often than women, and males aged 65 and over have the highest suicide rate in the United States.

Most people who commit suicide have given a specific verbal or nonverbal warning. It is not true that "anyone who talks about suicide doesn't do it."

Suicide may be the culmination of self-destructive tendencies that result from the client's turning his or her anger inward. The client may be asking for help by attempting suicide. Depressed clients may certainly be suicidal, but not all suicidal clients are depressed.

The risk of suicide is increased:

—when a plan is formulated
—when attempts become more painful or more violent
—when the client is male, adolescent, or over 45 years old
—when the client is divorced, widowed, separated, or living without family
—when the client gives away personal possessions, settles accounts, "ties up loose ends," and so forth
—when the client is in an early stage of treatment with antidepressant medications and his or her mood and activity level begin to elevate
—when the client's mood or activity level suddenly changes.

The specific actions or precautions taken by the nursing staff to protect a client from suicidal gestures or attempts vary with the client's individual needs (see the "Nursing Objectives and Nursing Actions" section). Many inhospital suicides occur during times that are unstructured and during which there are few staff.

There may be legal ramifications associated with the suicidal client who is hospitalized, especially if the client does commit suicide. It is especially important to observe the client and record his or her behavior carefully in the chart and to communicate *any* pertinent information to others who are making decisions about the client (especially if the client is to go on activities, on pass, or to be discharged).

Remember: Threatening suicide may be an effort to bring about a fundamental change in the client's life situation or elicit a response from a significant person. *Remember*: Every client has the potential for suicide.

BEHAVIORS OR PROBLEMS

Suicidal ideation, rumination, or plans
Self-destructive tendencies
Suicidal gestures or attempts
Low self-esteem
Feelings of worthlessness
Lack of future orientation
Lack of impulse control
Problems of depression, substance abuse, personality disorder, behavioral disorder, or other psychiatric problems (see other care plans as appropriate)

SHORT-TERM GOALS

Provide a safe environment for the client.
Prevent injury to the client.
Facilitate the appropriate expression of feelings (especially guilt and anger).

LONG-TERM GOALS

Increase the client's feelings of self-worth and self-esteem.

Assist the client to acknowledge and accept feelings of anger toward others, and any other feelings that may be unacceptable to the client.

Increase the client's insight into his or her behavior.

Increase the client's ability to deal with his or her feelings without using suicidal behavior.

Increase the client's impulse control.

Increase the client's ability to deal with suicidal feelings and urges after discharge (see Care Plan 2, Discharge Planning).

NURSING OBJECTIVES	NURSING ACTIONS
Provide a safe environment, and protect the client from self-destructive tendencies. Decrease suicidal behavior.	Determine the appropriate level of suicide precautions for the client. Institute these precautions immediately upon admission (may be by nursing order or by physician's order). Some suggested levels of suicide precautions are: 1. The client has one-to-one contact with a staff member at all times, even when going to the bathroom. The client is restricted to the unit and can use nothing that may be used to harm self (e.g., sharp objects, belt). 2. The client has one-to-one contact with a staff member at all times, but may attend activities off the unit (maintaining one-to-one contact). 3. Special attention: the client's whereabouts and activities should be known at all times on the unit. The client must be accompanied by a staff member while off the unit, but may be in a staff-client group. Assess the client's suicidal potential and evaluate the level of suicide precautions daily. In your initial assessment, note any previous suicide attempts and methods, as well as family history of mental illness or suicide. Obtain this information in a matter-of-fact manner; do not discuss in length or dwell on details. Ask the client if he or she has a plan for suicide. Attempt to ascertain how detailed and how feasible the plans are. *Remember*: As depression lessens, the client may have the energy to carry out a plan for suicide. Explain suicide precautions to the client.

NURSING OBJECTIVES (Continued)	NURSING ACTIONS (Continued)
	Be especially alert to sharp objects and other potentially dangerous items (e.g., glass containers, glass ashtrays, vases, matches, cigarettes); these items should not be in the client's possession.
	The client's room should be centrally located, preferably near the nurses' station within view of the staff. Avoid rooms at the end of a hallway or near the exit, elevator, or stairwell.
	Make sure the windows are locked such that the client cannot open them (in a general hospital the maintenance department may have to seal the windows).
	If it is necessary for the client to use sharp objects, sign out all sharps to the client and stay with the client during their use. Have the client use an electric shaver if possible.
	It may be necessary to restrain the client or to place him or her in seclusion with no objects that can be used to self-inflict injury (e.g., electrical outlets, silverware, even bedclothing).
Maintain close supervision of the client.	Know the whereabouts of the client at all times. Designate a specific staff person to be responsible for the client at all times. If this person must leave the unit, information and responsibility regarding supervision of the client must be transferred to another staff person.
	Stay with the client when he or she is meeting hygienic needs such as bathing, shaving, cutting nails, etc.
	Check the client at frequent, *irregular* intervals during the night to ascertain the client's safety and whereabouts.
	Maintain especially close supervision of the client at any time there is a decrease in the number of staff, decrease in the amount of structure or in the level of stimulation (e.g., nursing report at the change of shift, mealtime, weekends, nights). Also be especially aware of the client during any period of turmoil or distraction and when clients are going to or from activities.

NURSING OBJECTIVES (Continued)	NURSING ACTIONS (Continued)
	Observe the client and note behavior patterns; use this information to plan nursing care and the client's activities (for example, when is the client more animated? withdrawn?). Note behaviors with regard to the time of day, structured versus unstructured time, interactions with others, tasks, activities, responsibilities, and attention span.
	Be aware of the relationships the client is forming with other clients. Note who may become his or her confidant (whom the client may warn about a suicide attempt), and any manipulative or attention-seeking behavior.
	Be alert to the possibility of the client saving up his or her own medications or obtaining medicines or dangerous objects from other clients or visitors.
	Note: The client may ask you "not to tell anyone" something the client may tell you. Avoid promising the client confidentiality in this way; make it clear to the client that you must share all information with the other staff members on the treatment team, but assure the client of confidentiality with regard to anyone outside the treatment team.
Be alert to possible signs that might lead to suicidal behavior.	Observe, record, and report any changes in the client's mood (e.g., elation, withdrawal, sudden resignation).
	Watch for such behavior patterns as: decreased communication; conversations about death or the futility of life; disorientation; low frustration tolerance; dependency and dissatisfaction with dependence; disinterest in surroundings; concealing articles which could be used to harm self.
Decrease rumination or excessive talk about suicide.	Tell the client that while you are willing to discuss emotions or other topics, you will not discuss prior suicide attempts or details of them repeatedly. (Discourage such conversations with other clients also.)
Increase feelings of self-worth.	Convey that you care about the client and that you believe the client is a worthwhile human being.

NURSING OBJECTIVES *(Continued)*	NURSING ACTIONS *(Continued)*
	Encourage the client to ventilate his or her feelings; convey your acceptance of the client's feelings. Do not joke about death, belittle the client's wishes or feelings, or make insensitive remarks such as "Everybody really wants to live." Do not belittle the client's prior suicide attempts, which other staff members may deem "only gestures." Persons who make suicidal gestures are gambling with death and need help.
	Provide opportunities for the client to succeed and give positive feedback for even very "small" accomplishments. *Note*: The client's self-esteem may be so low that the client may feel able, for example, to make things only for others at first, not for personal use.
	Help the client identify positive aspects about himself or herself, other people, his or her vocation, life situation, etc.
	Involve the client as much as possible in planning his or her treatment.
Decrease withdrawal; increase communication with others.	Convey your interest in the client. Seek out the client for interaction at least once per shift.
	If the client says, "I don't feel like talking," "I don't want to talk to you," "Leave me alone," etc., either remain with the client in silence (conveying interest and caring), or state that you will be back later to talk or be with the client, and withdraw. You may tell the client that you will return at a certain time.
	Give the client support for efforts to remain out of his or her room, to interact with other clients, or to attend activities.
	See Care Plan 9, Depression.
Help the client develop insight and increase ability to express and deal with his or her feelings in a healthy manner.	Encourage and support the client's expression of anger. (*Remember*: Do not take the anger personally.) Help the client deal with the fear of expressing anger, the fear of subsequent consequences and feelings, and so forth. Encourage the client to express fears and ventilate feelings; support the client in expressing anger or making

plans to directly express anger when it occurs. Help the client identify situations in which he or she would feel more comfortable expressing feelings; use role-playing to practice the expression of anger.

Provide opportunities for the client to express feelings and release tension in a healthy way.

With the client, examine the client's relationships outside the hospital: Is any person or group reinforcing the client's suicidal behavior? (Family therapy may be indicated.)

See Care Plan 25, Passive-Aggressive or Manipulative Behavior.

Do not make moral judgments about suicide, or reinforce the client's feelings of guilt or sin.

Attempt to alleviate anxiety related to the client's religious concerns (e.g., feelings about guilt, death, suicide, etc.).

If possible, contact a chaplain or other member of the clergy to talk with the client.

Help the client prepare for discharge; increase the client's ability to deal with possible suicidal feelings or urges that arise in the future.

Remember: Because the client is no longer suicidal, it does not mean the client is ready for discharge.

Discuss the future with the client; consider hypothetical situations, emotional concerns, significant relationships, and future plans.

Plan out with the client how he or she will deal with feelings and situations that have precipitated suicidal feelings or behavior in the past. Include whom the client will contact (ideally identify someone in the home environment), where to go, what things may alleviate suicidal feelings (what has worked in the past). Also include how to recognize the building up of such feelings and deal with them before the client reaches a critical point.

Examine the client's home environment. What, if any, changes should occur to decrease the likelihood of suicidal behavior?

See Care Plan 2, Discharge Planning.

Grief Reaction

The normal grief process has been described as consisting of several stages, including denial, anger, ambivalence, acceptance, and integration of the experience into plans for the future. This progression is not necessarily in a certain order; moreover, "skipping" stages is common, and the time spent in each phase and in the process as a whole varies considerably among individuals (from weeks to years). The client must actually work through these phases, expressing and accepting the feelings involved (although all of this work may not be done in the hospital).

Grief can be for the loss of anything significant to the client, such as: health (upon learning of illness, or after sudden injury or disability), a job, a pet, a loved one (through death or other termination of the relationship), a role (e.g., the mother role when the youngest child grows up and leaves home). Grief work can be delayed for an indefinite time and may be the source of or a factor in another illness.

Discharge planning is extremely important with an adaptation of the client's lifestyle to the loss (new life situation); also new methods of dealing with stress must be developed (especially if the lost person or object was integral to previous coping strategies).

Loss and grief work are significant stresses from which the client must recuperate physically as well as emotionally; rest, exercise, nutrition, hydration, and elimination should be encouraged during hospitalization and as part of the discharge plans. The goal in grief work is *not* to avoid or eliminate painful feelings. Rather, it is to experience, express, work through, and be comfortable with even these "negative" emotions.

BEHAVIORS OR PROBLEMS

Difficulty in accepting significant loss
Denial of loss
Denial of feelings (flat affect)
Ambivalent feelings toward lost object
Guilt feelings
Inability to express feelings
Rumination
Fear of intensity of feelings
Depressive symptoms (e.g., withdrawn behavior) (see Care Plan 9, Depression)
Suicidal ideation (see Care Plan 10, Suicidal Behavior)

SHORT-TERM GOALS

Identify the loss.
Express feelings.
Decrease guilt.
Decrease suicidal ideation and depressive symptoms.
Progress through the phases of grief reaction.
Recuperate from the stress of loss.

LONG-TERM GOALS

Accept the loss.
Integrate the loss into the client's life.
Adapt lifestyle incorporating the fact of the loss.
Develop new coping strategies.
Make future plans with integration of the loss (see Care Plan 2, Discharge Planning).

NURSING OBJECTIVES	NURSING ACTIONS
Establish rapport (build trust) so the client feels comfortable expressing feelings which may be difficult to accept or express.	At first assign the same staff members to the client to develop trust and promote consistency. Then vary the staff persons to prevent an undue dependence on certain staff members and to promote client's comfort in expressing feelings to others.
Facilitate the client's progression through the stages of grieving. Decrease the fear of being overwhelmed by feelings and the fear of feelings as destructive, harmful, and to be pushed away.	Discourage rumination or stopping in one stage of grief work (i.e., if the client is ruminating on his or her own guilt, for example, after listening to the client's feelings, tell the client you will talk about other aspects of grief and feelings).
	Discourage the client's use of hospitalization or activities as avoidance of grief work ("to get my mind off it").
	Convey to the client that although feelings are uncomfortable, they are natural and necessary to this process, that the client can withstand having these feelings, and that the client will not be harmed by them.
	Point out to the client that this is a nurturing time, a time of learning and growth from which to gather the strength to go forward.
	Convey that although the client does not have to think or talk about his or her feelings at all times, a part of each day should be spent dealing with or being aware of them. Talk with the client at least once per shift about his or her loss, feelings, plans, etc.
Decrease denial; help the client grasp the fact of the loss.	After establishing rapport with the client, bring up the loss in a supportive manner; if the client refuses to discuss it, withdraw and state your intention to return ("I can understand that you may not want to talk with me about this now. I will come to talk with you again at 11:00; maybe we can talk about it then."). Do return at the stated time; then continue to be as supportive as possible rather than confrontative.
	Talk with the client in realistic terms concerning his or her loss: discuss concrete situations or changes that have occurred in his or her life as a result of the loss, and changes that the client must now begin to make, etc.

NURSING OBJECTIVES (Continued)	NURSING ACTIONS (Continued)
Encourage identification of the loss and the expression of feelings about the lost object or person and the client's relationship with the object or person.	Encourage the expression of feelings in ways with which the client is comfortable: verbal, written, drawing, crying, etc. Convey your acceptance of these feelings and means of expression.
	Encourage the client to recall experiences, talk about what was involved in his or her relationship with the lost object or person, and so forth.
	Note: If you feel uncomfortable with the client's expression of feelings (crying), or uncomfortable bringing up painful feelings, then withdraw temporarily, examine and try to become comfortable with your own feelings or have the client speak to someone who is comfortable.
Facilitate the client's expression of ambivalent or angry feelings toward the lost object or person (e.g., anger, hatred, resentment of grief work and the energy it takes, feelings of being deserted) and toward self. Work through feelings of guilt and betrayal.	Encourage appropriate (i.e., safe) expression of all feelings that the client has toward the lost object or person and convey acceptance (it may be appropriate to assure the client that even "negative" feelings are "normal" and healthy in grieving). Provide opportunities for the release of tension and guilt through physical activities. (Also promote regular physical exercise as a healthy continuing means of expression of and dealing with stress, tension, etc.)
Discourage the client's dependence on a particular staff member (or on the hospital) for expression of feelings. Decrease secondary gain from depression. Facilitate growth in ability to express and deal with feelings (in or out of the hospital). Encourage early discharge planning.	Limit times and frequency of therapeutic interactions with the client. Encourage independent, spontaneous expression of feelings (e.g., writing, initiating interaction with other clients or with other staff members, physical activity). Plan staff-initiated interactions to allow the client to fulfill other responsibilities (e.g., activities, ward duties) and personal care (e.g., sleep, meals).
	Expect the client to fulfill his or her own responsibilities and support the client for doing so. Withdraw your attention when the client does not fulfill responsibilities (i.e., do not have therapeutic interaction when the client has refused to participate in an activity).
	As much as possible, include in each interaction with the client some discussion of goals, the future, and discharge plans (see Care Plan 2, Discharge Planning).

| --- | --- |
Encourage ventilation of feelings within the therapeutic milieu; facilitate a supportive environment for the client (such as the larger client group).	Encourage the client to talk with other clients, individually and in small groups (larger as tolerated) about the loss, in terms of his or her own and others' feelings, and experiences and changes incurred in life. Facilitate sharing, communication, ventilation of feelings, and support.
	Utilize larger groups (e.g., open report) for a general discussion of loss and grief (with or without focusing on this client) to facilitate communication, support, and sharing. However, help the client realize that there are limits in sharing—dwelling on grief alone can make other people uncomfortable and may lead to the client being avoided by friends and significant others.
Decrease depressive symptoms (i.e., loss of appetite, sleep disturbances, withdrawn behavior, and suicidal ideation).	See Care Plan 9, Depression, and Care Plan 10, Suicidal Behavior.
Encourage the client to explore emotional changes as a result of the loss.	Discuss with the client the changes in his or her feelings toward self, others, and the lost object or person.
Encourage the client to consciously adapt his or her lifestyle to the loss and make concrete and realistic future plans.	Help the client plan for the future with regard to changes made necessary by the loss, at whatever levels the loss affects (living arrangements, finances, social activities, vocation, recreation, etc.). Utilize hospital and community resources. (See Care Plan 2, Discharge Planning.)
Help the client recuperate from the stress caused by the loss (attain optimal level of health and functioning).	Point out to the client that a major aspect of loss is a real physical stress. Encourage (and monitor, if necessary) good nutrition, hydration, and elimination, as well as adequate rest and daily physical exercise (recreational such as walking, running, swimming, cycling, etc.).
	Also urge the client (and facilitate) to identify and pursue his or her own strengths inside and outside the hospital to help balance painful talks and to deal with continuing depression.

Altered Body Image

The client's perception of his or her altered body image is more significant than the concrete disability or loss. The intensity of the client's reactions or feelings is not necessarily proportional to the actual loss or disability. The removal of an internal portion of the body may be as significant to the client as the loss of an extremity that is visible.

BEHAVIORS OR PROBLEMS

Feelings of anger, hostility, outrage
Depression (see Care Plan 9, Depression)
Feelings of hopelessness, worthlessness
Withdrawn behavior
Self-destructive behavior
Alienation from family or friends
Refusal to perform activities of daily living when physically capable
Identity concerns (sexual, role as breadwinner or parent, etc.)

SHORT-TERM GOALS

Identify the disability or loss.
Ventilate feelings (e.g., anger, hostility).
Clarify the client's perception of altered body image.
Increase feelings of self-worth.
Prevent self-destructive behavior (see Care Plan 10, Suicidal Behavior).

LONG-TERM GOALS

Resolve grief or loss.
Adapt lifestyle to accommodate the disability or loss.

Care Plans Related to Physical Symptoms

Clients may manifest various physical symptoms that are related to emotional or psychiatric problems. Although these symptoms may or may not have a demonstrable organic cause, they are nevertheless quite real to the client and should not be minimized or dismissed. The care plans in this section differentiate the kinds of problems encountered in these situations as well as give suggestions for use in an individual care plan.

It is important to remember that because a client has emotional problems, not all of the physical complaints that the client voices are necessarily caused by or related to those problems. A client's complaint or perception should never be disregarded because he or she is "just faking it," or because he or she has made many complaints. Also, some physical problems do indeed have a base in organic physiology as well as in stress or emotional difficulties (psychosomatic illnesses). Other behaviors or problems do not have a demonstrable organic cause, but are real to the client and must be treated as such (hypochondriacal behavior). Finally, symptoms may be due to an unconscious process through which the client is attempting to deal with a conflict (conversion reaction) and, again, these symptoms are very real to the client.

As in other sections in this book, the care plans in this section deal with those problems and behaviors primarily related to physical symptoms. Other care plans may also be appropriate in planning care with the individual client whose major problem is described here.

Psychosomatic Disorders

The term *psychosomatic* is from the Greek words *psyche*, meaning mind, and *soma*, meaning body. The client may be experiencing a common physical illness, which the client or the therapist may see as having been caused by or exacerbated by stress or emotional illness. These physical difficulties, which may be construed as having psychosomatic components or origins, may involve any organ system. Some commonly accepted examples of this are: psoriasis, ulcers, ulcerative colitis, headaches, rheumatoid arthritis, asthma, hyperventilation, palpitations, and anorexia nervosa.

Theories on psychosomatic illness range from the belief that all physical problems are "organic" in nature, having nothing to do with the psyche, to the belief that all physical problems are manifestations of or result from emotional ills. Theories also vary with regard to how symptoms or disease states are related to a particular emotional problem. Certain "target organs" may be seen as symbolic of the client's anxieties or stresses, or the client may be considered to subconsciously direct stress to those body parts. Or, perhaps the target organ was genetically weak in the client and therefore it reacts with extra sensitivity to stress or anxiety.

Psychosomatic disorders are distinct from hypochondriacal behavior in that they are *real* physical diseases or symptom complexes with organic pathology that have their bases in life stresses or psychiatric problems. Hypochondriacal disorders have no organic pathology. (See Care Plan 13, Hypochondriacal Behavior.) Psychosomatic disorders may result in structural or organic changes in the body and may become life-threatening illnesses.

BEHAVIORS OR PROBLEMS

Physical complaints, symptoms, or disease complex(es)
Resistance to the role of a psychiatric client or to therapy
Denial of emotional problems or stress
Anxiety, fear
Anger or hostility (see Care Plan 23, Hostility)
Resentment, guilt
Low self-esteem
Depression (see Care Plan 9, Depression)
High level of stress in life
Dependency needs (see Care Plan 26, Dependency or Inadequacy)
Secondary gain (e.g., attention, evasion of responsibilities) due to illness (see Care Plan 25, Passive-Aggressive or Manipulative Behavior)

SHORT-TERM GOALS

Successfully treat acute physical problems (actual physical condition).
Incorporate the client in planning care.
Accept the treatment plan.
Decrease denial of emotional problems.
Recognize feelings of stress, anxiety, anger, and other related feelings.
Increase ability to express feelings.
Decrease anxiety.
Increase willingness to relinquish the "sick role."
Examine the client's life situation; identify stresses and their relationship to disease.

Develop insight.
Decrease secondary gain.

LONG-TERM GOALS

Increase insight.
Increase self-esteem.

Increase ability to express feelings.
Develop alternative ways to deal with life stresses and the anxiety or other feelings they may cause.
Eliminate secondary gain.
Achieve physical health or the management of the disorder.

NURSING OBJECTIVES	NURSING ACTIONS
Accurately assess and treat the client's acute physical problems (actual physical condition).	In the initial interview, do a thorough systems review for physical problems, complaints, history of diseases, treatment, surgeries, or hospitalizations. *Remember*: The client may attempt to minimize or maximize his or her physical problems.
	Develop a nursing care plan regarding the client's physical health and implement it as soon as possible. Be matter-of-fact in your approach and treatment. Do not overemphasize physical problems or care, but remember that the client's problems are physically real and not hypochondriacal (i.e., imaginary) in nature.
Incorporate the client in planning his or her care. Gain the client's acceptance of the treatment plan.	Talk with the client honestly regarding a possible correlation between emotions or stress and physical symptoms or disease states.
	Ask for the client's perceptions regarding his or her hospitalization and physical problems. However, do not argue with the client or put the client on the defensive.
	Ask what the client's expectations are of the hospital stay, both of self and the hospital staff. Try to involve the client in care planning, identifying problems, setting goals, and choosing actions to work toward those goals. See Care Plan 1, Building a Trust Relationship.
Identify feelings of stress, anxiety, and related feelings. Increase ability to express feelings.	Assess the client's lifestyle (activities and interactions with others) with regard to stress, support systems, dependency needs, and expression of emotions.
Decrease denial. Increase insight. Decrease anxiety and anger.	Talk with the client about your observations and assessment. Ask for the client's perceptions regarding stress, sources of satisfaction and dissatisfaction in his or her daily life, significant relationships, work, etc.

	If the client denies that he or she experiences stress or certain feelings, the discussion may need to be less direct. For example, point out possible or apparent stresses or feelings of the client and ask the client for feedback.
	Without always connecting the client's physical problems with the client's emotions, encourage the client to identify and express feelings to self (e.g., in writing), to staff members (in individual conversations), and in groups (small, informal, progressing to larger and more formal).
	Gradually, with the client, attempt to identify the connections between anxiety or stress and the exacerbation of the client's physical problems.
Increase self-esteem.	Provide activities that the client can easily accomplish at first, such as simple tasks with which the client is already familiar, or which the client can complete in a short time (e.g., 15 to 20 minutes). Gradually introduce the client to more complex, challenging, or competitive activities.
	Give the client direct positive feedback for accomplishments and fulfillment of responsibilities. Do not flatter the client or be otherwise dishonest.
	It may be helpful for the client to identify his or her own strengths (e.g., make a written list).
	See Care Plan 9, Depression, and Care Plan 1, Building a Trust Relationship.
Decrease secondary gains.	Talk with the client and his or her significant others regarding the concept of secondary gains and together develop a plan to: —identify the needs the client is attempting to meet (e.g., need for attention, means of dealing with perceived excess responsibilities or with stress); —attempt to meet these needs in more direct ways.
	Individual conferences with the client's family or significant others may be helpful in identifying their attitudes and behaviors. For example, they may unknowingly be giving the client the message that emotional problems are a sign of weakness, and that only physical illness is acceptable.

NURSING OBJECTIVES *(Continued)*	NURSING ACTIONS *(Continued)*
Develop alternative ways to deal with feelings and stress.	Encourage the client to continue to identify stresses after his or her discharge from the hospital and to attempt to deal with them directly.
	Support the client's continued ventilation of feelings and encourage the client to develop an outside support system for this (e.g., with significant others, with an ongoing support group, or through group therapy if indicated).
	Especially support the client for spontaneous or unsolicited expression of feelings, or for ventilation of feelings independent of others (e.g., through writing, artwork).
	Encourage the client to identify and express his or her feelings directly in interpersonal relationships and stressful situations—especially feelings with which the client has been uncomfortable. You might let the client role play situations within a group and support his or her successful expression of feelings.
	Encourage the client to modify his or her lifestyle to enhance health (e.g., with regular exercise, good nutrition).
	See Care Plan 2, Discharge Planning.

Hypochondriacal Client

The client may feel real symptoms (e.g., pain), even though an organic basis for the symptoms cannot be found. It is important to carefully assess the client's physical condition and to refer somatic complaints (at least the first time the client makes the specific complaint) to the medical staff for evaluation; do *not* assume a complaint is hypochondriacal until after this evaluation.

The client may be successfully avoiding certain responsibilities (vocational, educational, familial), receiving attention, or manipulating others by exhibiting symptoms or expressing complaints. This is called *secondary gain*. It may be helpful to work with the client's family or significant others to decrease or eliminate secondary gains and develop healthy ways for the client to receive attention, deal with responsibilities, and so on.

Somatic complaints may be a mechanism that the client has learned to use as a way to deal with feelings, anxieties, or conflicts; the client may not be able to relinquish this behavior until the anxiety decreases or other behaviors develop (see also Care Plan 27, Obsessive Thoughts or Compulsive Behavior). Hypochondriacal symptoms may be found in clients having difficulty expressing anger satisfactorily, including clients with several types of psychiatric disorders, such as depression, schizophrenia, neurosis, or personality disorders. The client may be using denial mechanisms and attempting (subconsciously) to turn emotions (e.g., anger) into physical ailments.

These clients can be very frustrating to work with. It is important to identify and work through personal feelings that arise while working with them. The prognosis is often poor because of their pattern of dissatisfaction with and rejection of treatment (changing physicians or hospitals), denial of feelings, or other neurotic patterns.

BEHAVIORS OR PROBLEMS

Denial of emotional problems

Difficulty identifying and expressing feelings

Self-preoccupation, especially with physical functioning

Fears of or rumination on disease

Numerous somatic complaints—may involve many different organs or systems

Sensory complaints (e.g., loss of taste sensation, olfactory complaints)

Reluctance or refusal to participate in psychiatric treatment program or activities

Reliance on medications or physical treatments (e.g., laxative dependence)

Extensive use of over-the-counter medications, home remedies, enemas, etc.

History of repeated visits to physicians or hospital admissions

History of repeated medical work-ups with no findings of abnormalities

Secondary gains (attention, evasion of responsibilities) due to "ailments"

Fatigue

Insomnia

Anxiety

Loss of appetite

Weight changes

Tremors

Ritualistic behaviors (e.g., exaggerated bowel routines) (see Care Plan 27, Obsessive Thoughts or Compulsive Behavior)

Delusions (see Care Plan 6, Delusions)

SHORT-TERM GOALS

Accurately assess and treat somatic complaints.

Minimize the time and attention given to physical complaints.

Decrease the number and frequency of physical and sensory complaints.

Decrease or eliminate rumination, excessive fears of disease, and delusions.

Help the client identify his or her life stresses and anxieties, and relate them to somatic complaints.

Increase ability to express feelings.

Decrease secondary gains.

Increase participation in treatment program.

Decrease reliance on and use of medications and physical treatments.

Decrease fatigue, anorexia, anxiety, insomnia, or tremors.

Decrease ritualistic behaviors.

LONG-TERM GOALS

Eliminate physical complaints.

Increase insight into behavior and the dynamics of the disorder.

Eliminate other symptoms (e.g., fatigue, anorexia).

Eliminate ritualistic behaviors.

Decrease or eliminate overuse of medications or physical treatments.

Develop alternative ways to deal with stress or anxiety.

NURSING OBJECTIVES	NURSING ACTIONS
Accurately assess and treat somatic complaints.	The initial nursing assessment should include a complete review of organ systems, a history of previous complaints and treatment, and consideration of each present complaint.
	The nursing staff should note the medical staff's assessment of each complaint on the client's admission.
	Each time the client voices a new complaint (or claims injury), the client should be referred to the medical staff for assessment. *Remember*: Do not assume that all of the client's complaints are hypochondriacal in nature.
Decrease the number and frequency of physical and sensory complaints.	Minimize the amount of time and attention given to complaints. When the client makes a complaint, refer him or her to the medical staff (if it is a new complaint) or follow the team treatment plan; then tell the client that you will discuss something else, but not bodily complaints. Tell the client that you are interested in the client as a person, not just in his or her physical complaints (if the complaint is not acute, ask the client to save the complaint until a regular appointment with the medical staff).
	Withdraw your attention if the client insists on making complaints the sole topic of conversation. Tell the client your reason for withdrawal and that you desire to discuss other topics or interact at a later time.
	Allow the client a specific time period (e.g., 5 minutes per hour), to discuss physical complaints

with one person. The remaining staff will discuss only other issues with the client.

Remember: Do not argue with the client about his or her somatic complaints. Acknowledge the complaint as the client's feeling and then follow the above approaches.

Decrease rumination, delusions, and excessive fears of disease.

Decrease ritualistic behaviors.

Use the actions suggested above, as well as minimal objective reassurance in conjunction with questions (or other techniques) to explore the client's feelings (e.g., "Your tests have shown that you have no lesions. Do you still feel that you do? What are your feelings about this?").

Encourage the client to discuss his or her feelings about the fears (not the fears themselves).

See also Care Plan 6, Delusions, and Care Plan 27, Obsessive Thoughts or Compulsive Behavior.

Help the client identify life stresses and problems. Increase his or her insight into the disorder. Increase the client's expression of feelings.

Initially, carefully assess the client's self-image, social patterns, ways of dealing with anger, stress, and so forth.

Talk with the client about his or her daily life, family and other significant relationships, work, sources of satisfaction and dissatisfaction.

After some discussion of the above and the continued strengthening of a trust relationship, talk more directly with the client and encourage the client to talk openly about specific stresses, recent and ongoing. What does the client perceive as stressful?

If the client is using denial as a defense mechanism, the discussion of stresses may need to be less direct, with the staff member pointing out apparent, probable, or possible stresses (in a nonthreatening way), and asking for the client's feedback.

Gradually, try to identify possible connections between stress or anxiety and the occurrence or exacerbation of physical symptoms. Points you might assess are: What makes the client more comfortable? Less comfortable? What is the client doing or what is going on around the client when he or she feels more or less comfortable or is experiencing symptoms?

The client can also keep a diary of events or situations, stresses, and occurrence of symptoms. This diary can then be used to point out relationships between stresses and symptoms.

Talk with the client at least once per shift, focusing on the identification of and expression of the client's feelings; encourage the client to ventilate feelings—verbally, by crying, in physical activities, etc.

Decrease secondary gains.

Talk with the client and the client's family or significant others about the concept of secondary gains, and together develop a plan to:

—identify the needs the client is attempting to meet with secondary gains (such as attention, escape from perceived excess responsibilities or from stress);

—attempt to meet these needs in more direct ways: for example, give the client attention when he or she is *not* exhibiting symptoms or complaints, give the client support for dealing with responsibilities directly or for asserting himself or herself in the face of stress or discomfort;

—reduce the "benefits" of illness as much as possible; for example, do not allow the client to avoid responsibilities by voicing somatic discomfort (do not excuse the client from activities, do not allow special privileges such as staying in bed, or dressing in night clothes).

Decrease reliance on and use of medications and physical treatments.

Develop alternative ways of dealing with stress and anxiety.

Work with the medical staff to limit the number, variety, strength, and frequency of medications, enemas, and so forth, that are made available to the client.

When the client requests a medication or treatment for a complaint, encourage the client to identify what precipitated the complaint, and to deal with the discomfort in other ways.

Observe and record the circumstances surrounding the occurrence or exacerbation of complaints; talk about your observations with the client.

Assist the client to identify and use nonchemical methods of pain relief such as relaxation techniques.

Teach the client more healthful daily living habits in regard to diet, sleep, comfort measures (for example, conscious relaxation techniques), adequate fluid intake, adequate program of daily exercise, the importance of decreased stimuli, rest, possible connection between caffeine and anxiety, and so forth.

Encourage the client to identify and express feelings directly in interpersonal relationships or stressful situations, especially those feelings with which the client is uncomfortable, such as anger or resentment.

Notice the client's interactions with others (clients, staff members, visitors, significant others, yourself) and give positive feedback for the direct expression of feelings, self-assertion, and especially for the expression of anger, resentment, and other so-called negative emotions.

Conversion Reaction

Conversion reactions are not within the conscious control of the client—he or she is not "faking" the physical symptom. Common sensory symptoms include impaired vision, blindness, deafness, and loss of sensation of the extremities. Common motor symptoms include mutism, paralysis of the extremities, dizziness, and ataxia. The physical symptom is directly related to the underlying conflict.

The physical symptom may give the client a legitimate reason to avoid the conflict. For example: A young man wishes to attend college, but his father wants him to remain at home to help him farm. The young man develops a paralysis of his legs, thereby rendering him unable to do farm work. His conflict is resolved by a physical disability beyond his control.

The physical symptom may represent "deserved punishment" for guilt feelings. For example: A young woman gains pleasure from seeing movies and watching television, which are specifically forbidden by her family's religious beliefs. She feels guilty because she has violated those beliefs and develops blindness as her punishment, which relieves the guilt.

The physical symptom is very real—the client actually cannot see or walk. The focus of therapeutic intervention, however, is on the resolution of the conflict and conflicting feelings, rather than on the physical symptom, per se. Removal from the conflict (e.g., hospitalization) frequently produces gradual relief or remission of the physical symptom. As the client approaches discharge, the physical symptom may return.

The conversion reaction is classified as a type of hysterical reaction. Therefore the client may experience other similar problems. (See Care Plan 28, Hysterical Behavior.)

BEHAVIORS OR PROBLEMS

Physical limitation or disability (e.g., blindness, paralysis, loss of voice)
Feelings of guilt, anxiety, or frustration
Indifference or lack of concern regarding the severity of the physical symptom
Low self-esteem
Difficulty handling anger, frustration, or conflict
Feelings of inadequacy
Development of secondary gain from the physical symptom

SHORT-TERM GOALS

Relieve acute stress or conflict.
Determine the basis of the physical symptom (organic causes must be ruled out by the physician or diagnostic tests).
Identify the underlying conflict.
Ventilate feelings of fear, guilt, or inadequacy.
Prevent secondary gain from the physical symptom.

LONG-TERM GOALS

Resolve the conflict producing the physical symptom.
Develop methods other than conversion of satisfactorily coping with conflict.
Avoid recurrence of the conversion reaction after discharge from the hospital.

NURSING OBJECTIVES	NURSING ACTIONS
Identify the source of conflict or stress.	Obtain the client's thorough history on admission. Contact his or her family or significant others if necessary to complete the history. Send for records from prior hospitalizations, if possible.
	Talk with the client about his or her life, what is important to the client, his or her usual environment, work, significant others, etc.
Determine the basis of the symptom.	Observe the client carefully when the symptom occurs, or if the symptom is constant, observe the client's behavior in general, especially in relation to the symptom. Document all observations, including precipitating events, if any, effects of the environment (e.g., the presence of others), and recovery.
	The physician may order various tests to rule out a physical (organic) basis of the symptom. Assist or prepare the client as necessary.
Relieve stress or conflict.	Hospitalization itself may relieve the conflict a great deal by removing the client from his or her usual environment. If the stress is in relation to a particular person (or persons) in the client's life, visits from that person or persons may need to be discouraged, restricted, or prevented.
Diminish the client's focus on the physical symptom.	Involve the client in the usual activities, self-care, eating in the dining room, and so on, as you would other clients.
Prevent secondary gain from the symptom.	Expect the client's participation. Make your expectations clear to the client. Do not give the client special privileges or excuse him or her from the expectations due to physical limitations. Do not argue with the client; withdraw your attention if necessary. (See also Care Plan 25, Passive-Aggressive or Manipulative Behavior.)
Maintain adequate nutrition, hydration, and elimination. Promote adequate rest and exercise. Prevent injury.	Assess the client's food and fluid intake, elimination, and amount of rest as unobtrusively as possible, to minimize the physical aspects of the client's problem.
	Any intervention regarding the client's physical status (poor food or fluid intake, lack of sleep, etc.) must be planned by the treatment team. All

NURSING OBJECTIVES (*Continued*)	**NURSING ACTIONS** (*Continued*)
	staff members must be unified and consistent in their approach.
	Supervise the client from a distance for the ability to perform activities of daily living, ambulate independently, and so on. Intervene if the client is risking injury to self, but minimize the attention given to the client's physical supervision.
	Remember: Usually clients with hysterical types of behavior will not experience physical harm, injury, or deprivation.
Encourage ventilation of feelings and a discussion of the conflict.	Focus nursing interactions on discussions of the client's feelings, his or her home or work situation, and relationships with others.
Facilitate recognition of the relationship between the conflict and the physical symptom.	Avoid long discussions of the physical symptom; withdraw your attention from the client if necessary.
Help the client resolve the conflict, or deal with it in ways other than by producing physical symptoms.	Praise the client if and when he or she is able to discuss the physical symptom as a method used to cope with conflict.
	Explore alternative methods of expressing feelings and dealing with the identified conflict. Evaluate the effectiveness of the alternative methods.
	Give the client positive feedback for expressing his or her feelings.
	Encourage the client to identify some strategies to deal with or resolve the conflict. (Family therapy may be indicated.)
Prepare the client for discharge. Prevent recurrence of the conversion reaction after discharge.	See Care Plan 2, Discharge Planning.
	Help the client find a support system outside the hospital.
	Plan follow-up care as needed.

Care Plans Related to Eating

Since there may be many reasons why a client does not eat, the first care plan in this section addresses the general problems of the client who will not eat and includes specific suggestions for various problems and cross-references to other care plans that may be appropriate in planning individual client care (such as depression, delusions, and so forth). The second care plan gives information regarding a specific disorder related to not eating, anorexia nervosa. Again, different approaches are presented and the suggestions given are to be adapted to and incorporated in the individual client's care plan as appropriate.

Client Who Will Not Eat

Clients who will not eat may have the following behaviors or problems as concomitant results or causes of not eating:

Depression, grief
Withdrawn behavior
Confusion
Manic behavior
Self-destructive feelings or behaviors
Manipulative behavior
Delusions
Phobias
Guilt
Anorexia nervosa (see Care Plan 16, Anorexia Nervosa)

Physical problems that may be related:

Electrolyte imbalance
Inadequate nutrition, hydration
Poor dental or denture condition
Poor coordination

BEHAVIORS OR PROBLEMS

Refusal to eat
Difficulty swallowing
Weight loss
Malnutrition
Inadequate hydration, elimination
Starvation

SHORT-TERM GOALS

Prevent death by starvation.
Establish and maintain adequate nutrition, hydration, and elimination.
Promote weight gain.
Decrease related delusions, phobias, guilt, depression (see other care plans as appropriate).
Increase self-esteem.
Prevent secondary gain that the client obtains by not eating.

LONG-TERM GOALS

Establish regular, adequate, nutritional eating habits.
Develop non-food-related coping mechanisms.

NURSING OBJECTIVES	NURSING ACTIONS
Accurately assess the client's present physical and nutritional state and his or her recent and normal eating habits.	On the client's admission, do a thorough assessment (utilize physical assessment, client and family interviews), to obtain detailed information regarding the client's eating patterns, familiar or liked foods, snacks, special diet (religious, vegetarian), changes in regular habits, gastrointestinal (GI) complaints and disorders (validated?), circumstances that affect the client's appetite, and so forth.

NURSING OBJECTIVES *(Continued)*	NURSING ACTIONS *(Continued)*
Accurately observe and record the client's intake and output.	Strictly monitor intake and output. (Do not call the client's attention to intake and output notation; try to make unobtrusive observations.) Note and record: the type and amount of food, the times and circumstances of eating (was the client alone? was eating encouraged? what was the level of stimuli?).
	Weigh the client regularly (the client should wear only a hospital gown when weighed).
Promote adequate elimination.	Provide fruit juices and foods high in bulk.
	Keep a record of the client's bowel movements—their color, amount, consistency, and frequency. (*Remember:* if the client is consuming little or no food or liquids only, stools may be less frequent or loose.)
Increase the client's intake of food and liquids.	Have some food and liquids available at all times.
Maintain homeostasis.	Offer food, nutritious liquids, and water to the client frequently, in small amounts.
	Discourage the intake of nonnutritional substances (e.g., coffee), except water.
	Encourage the use of milk (rather than a nondairy creamer) in coffee or tea.
	Offer foods that require little effort to eat (i.e., easily chewed) and are visually pleasant.
	Encourage the intake of liquids highest in nutritional value and calories (e.g., orange juice is high in nutritive value; chocolate milk has 50 more calories per serving than white milk; whole milk can be ordered rather than skim or low-fat milk).
	Make high protein shakes available. They can be made from ice cream, milk, and powdered milk blended together (be sure to stir before giving to the client) or from dietary supplements (like fortified liquid meals or beverages).
	If the client has GI complaints (e.g., nausea), offer light, bland foods, clear soups, and clear carbonated beverages; avoid fried foods, gravy, or spicy foods.

NURSING OBJECTIVES (Continued)	NURSING ACTIONS (Continued)
	If the client will take only liquids, gradually attempt to introduce solid foods into his or her diet (begin with cream soups, crackers, light foods).
	Try to accommodate the client's normal or previous eating habits as much as possible.
	When offering foods, tell the client you have something for him or her to eat; do not ask if he or she wants to eat or feels like eating.
	It may be necessary to get food and feed the client; get food and offer to the client; accompany the client to get food; or sit with the client through mealtime. Nasogastric (NG) tube feedings or IV therapy may also be necessary.
	Do not tell the client that he or she will get sick, weak, or may die from not eating. Any of these may be the client's wish.
	Do not threaten the client, but do employ limits, consequences, consistency, and the giving or withdrawing of attention as appropriate (see Care Plan 16, Anorexia Nervosa).
Prevent secondary gain from not eating.	Give positive support and attention when the client eats; withdraw your attention when he or she refuses to eat.
Decrease manipulation of the staff.	Set up structured times and limits regarding eating (i.e., try to feed the client for 10 minutes, then withdraw for a half hour, etc.). Be consistent in your approach.
Establish or strengthen independent nutritional eating habits.	Gradually change from offering food to suggesting that the client get food for himself or herself. Observe and record changes in the frequency of eating and the amount eaten.
	Then gradually decrease the frequency of suggestions and allow the client to take the responsibility for eating; again record changes.
Develop non-food-related coping mechanisms.	Assess or explore the client's history, particularly his or her attitudes and feelings regarding food and eating (e.g., family emphasis on food, stress, pleasure, reward, guilt, resentment, religion, morality, control, and manipulation).
Decrease the association of food and not eating with guilt, depression, or punishment.	

Allow the client to have food only at specified snack times and mealtimes.

Encourage the client to ventilate his or her feelings at times other than mealtimes.

Observe and record the client's perceptions of and responses to stress; encourage the client to approach a staff member when experiencing stress.

Talk with the client to identify others in his or her environment with whom the client can talk, and what other activities may decrease stress or anxieties (e.g., hobbies, physical activities).

Discourage (withdraw your attention from) rituals (elaborate or otherwise) or emotional associations with meals, food, etc.

Anorexia Nervosa

The usual characteristics of anorexics consist of:

Pale, dry skin, poor skin turgor, little subcutaneous tissue
Above average intelligence
Middle- to upper-class socioeconomic level
Puritanical philosophy, high personal standards
Interested in food, cooking
Alert, cheerful, hyperactive
May have been overweight at one time, but not necessarily (*note:* anorexia is not always a "diet taken too far")
May have periods of rigid self-starvation without conscious hunger, alternating with periods of eating huge amounts of food without satiety
History of obsessional traits, early feeding difficulties, family emphasis on food or mealtimes (which are often emotional or stressful)
Physiological disturbances: abnormal GTT curve, increased serum cholesterol and carotene, decreased urinary 17-ketosteroids, estrogens, testosterone, and gonadotropins

Prognosis: Fifty percent fully recover; 10 to 15 percent die prematurely. Death occurs from starvation and complications. These clients develop psychoses no more often than the general population. The illness may be an attempt to control the person's life or body and achieve a sense of identity.

Disgust at the thought of eating
Preoccupation with food
Hiding and hoarding of food
Weight loss
Phobic concern with weight
Unceasing pursuit of thinness
Cheating on diet
Vomiting
Difficulty swallowing
Denial of illness
Denial of being too thin
Body image distortions (may be of delusional proportions)
Flat affect
Problems with identity or self-image
Feelings of worthlessness
Family problems
Manipulation of staff members, family, or other clients
Physical problems or changes: malnutrition, lanugo (soft body hair), amenorrhea, bradycardia, low basal metabolic rate, temperature, and blood pressure, constipation, poor muscle tone and function, secondary sexual characteristics absent
Gorging
Retaining feces and urine
Eating large amounts of salt
Concealing weights on body to increase weight (especially prior to being weighed)

BEHAVIORS OR PROBLEMS

Refusal to eat
Loss of appetite
Dislike of certain foods

SHORT-TERM GOALS

Prevent death.
Increase caloric and nutritional intake.
Promote weight gain.
Build a trust relationship.

Build self-esteem.

Help develop non-food-related coping mechanisms.

Promote health.

Prevent the manipulation of staff members.

Obtain accurate weights.

Increase social skills.

Maintain adequate elimination.

Prevent secondary gains from not eating.

LONG-TERM GOALS

Establish regular, adequate, independent, and nutritional eating habits.

Decrease associations between food and stress (and other emotions).

Develop non–food-related coping mechanisms.

Improve home environment (e.g., family problems).

Prepare for discharge (see Care Plan 2, Discharge Planning).

Note: The following care plan suggests in detail one type of nursing care approach which may be used with clients with anorexia nervosa, especially if the client's life is threatened. Another approach that may be used does not focus on foods or mealtimes, but only on weight. As weight is gained in accordance with the goals set (per individual client), the client gains privileges. If weight is lost, privileges are lost also. No attention would be given to intake or output (hence, this approach may not be used in severe, or life-threatening, cases). Goals are set in accordance with the treatment plan; for example, a weekend pass when the client weighs 90 pounds, discharge when the client weighs 95 pounds. This plan can be continued after discharge when follow-up care can include rehospitalization if the client's weight falls below a certain level. (If the client actually likes hospitalization, the plan may need to include nasogastric (NG) tube feedings, and so forth, for long-term care.)

NURSING OBJECTIVES	NURSING ACTIONS
Increase the client's nutritional and caloric intake.	If the client can select items on his or her diet, do not make low-calorie foods available.
	The client should have as few distractions (e.g., television, conversation) as possible during mealtimes.
	The client's mealtimes can be structured and limited in time (at a specific time, and for a specific duration such as 40 minutes).
	Tell the client when it is time to eat; present the food; state the limit on the mealtime.
	After this time (if the client does not eat the meal), the NG tube should be inserted and the client thus fed a specified amount of liquid diet. If an NG tube is not used, IV therapy may be indicated.
	Withdraw your attention during the mealtime if the client refuses to eat.
	Monitor the client's intake and output. (A record should be kept at the nursing station by the nursing staff. Observations should be done as unobtrusively as possible.)

NURSING OBJECTIVES *(Continued)*	NURSING ACTIONS *(Continued)*
	The client's diet should include finger foods (especially for snacks) and foods the client likes.
Maintain adequate elimination.	Monitor the client's elimination patterns.
	Diet should include sufficient bulk and adequate amounts of fluid.
Build trust; increase rapport with the nursing staff.	The physician may (should) insert the NG tube.
	The NG tube should be inserted immediately after time for eating is past, with no bargaining allowed.
	Insertion should be in a nonpunitive manner.
Prevent siphoning.	The NG tube should *not* be left in place after feeding and should be reinserted each time it is indicated.
Promote weight gain.	The client may be without privileges (such as use of the telephone, ability to leave the unit without the nursing staff, choice of extra snack foods, decreased time restriction on meals) on admission, with privileges granted as weight is gained.
	If a weight loss occurs, decrease privileges, examine the circumstances, explore the feelings that motivated the loss.
Obtain accurate weights.	Weigh the client daily before the morning meal.
	Weigh the client in his or her hospital gown only.
	Accompany the client to the bathroom, and so forth, to prevent disposal of food or concealing of weights in or on the body.
Maintain consistency of treatment.	One staff member per shift should have the final word on decisions, although other members can have input.
Prevent or decrease manipulation of the staff.	Set and maintain strict limits, especially regarding mealtimes, amounts of food, tube feedings, weighing, privileges, etc.
	Communicate the limits and the consequences of exceeding those limits to the client clearly and in a nonpunitive manner.

NURSING OBJECTIVES (*Continued*)	NURSING ACTIONS (*Continued*)
Increase self-esteem. Increase social skills. Decrease feelings of inadequacy.	Give the client positive support and praise for things well done.
	Foster successful experiences: arrange for the client to help other clients in specific ways; identify and utilize the client's strengths.
	Begin by offering the client small tasks and activities that are easily accomplished. Increase the tasks in complexity as appropriate.
	Focus attention on the client's positive traits and tasks accomplished (not on feelings of inadequacy).
	Utilize recreational or occupational therapy as appropriate.
	Staff members should remain aware of their function as role models (be consistent, observant, responsive, truthful, and empathetic).
Improve home environment. Increase the client's ability to function in his or her home environment.	Assess the client's home environment: interview the client's family; make a home visit if possible. Family therapy may be indicated. Encourage the family's participation in such therapy.
	Encourage the client to ventilate his or her feelings about family members, family dynamics, family roles, and so forth.
Decrease the association between food and stress.	Allow the client food only at specified snack times and mealtimes.
Help the client develop non–food-related coping mechanisms.	Encourage the client to ventilate his or her feelings.
	Observe and record the client's perceptions of and responses to stress; encourage the client to approach the staff at stressful times.
	Talk with the client to identify others in his or her environment with whom the client can talk, and what other activities may decrease stress or anxieties (e.g., hobbies, physical activities).
	Discourage (withdraw your attention from) rituals (elaborate or otherwise) or emotional associations with meals, food, etc.

NURSING OBJECTIVES *(Continued)*	NURSING ACTIONS *(Continued)*
Help the client to establish regular, adequate, independent, nutritional dietary habits.	Begin with strictly specified times for and limits on mealtimes and snack times.
	Assess the client's knowledge of nutrition and healthful dietary habits. Client teaching may be indicated (if this is done, it should be factual, unemotional, in concrete terms, and should also be limited in frequency and duration).
	Gradually increase the client's control over his or her food intake, choice, preparation, etc., as weight gain occurs.
Prepare the client for discharge and successful reintegration into home environment.	Discharge should not occur until the client reaches the "normal" weight for age and height. (See also Care Plan 2, Discharge Planning.)
	Send the client home for a specified time period, then evaluate the success of this in the hospital before discharging the client.
	Observe and record the client's feelings, mood, and activities before and after time at home.
	Involve the client's family with the client in teaching, treatment, and discharge and follow-up plans.
	Arrange for the client's follow-up care as appropriate.

Care Plans Related to Substance Abuse

Abuse of chemical substances may be chronic or acute, and it includes the use or abuse of alcohol, licit (prescription or over-the-counter drugs), or illicit drugs. The first two care plans in this section are concerned with the acute or short-term treatment plans for a client who is intoxicated or who is withdrawing from a chemical substance. Substance abuse involves definite physiological problems, often specific to the kind of substance used by the client, emotional difficulties, and may involve social, economic, vocational, and legal difficulties as well. The last care plan describes a possible program that can be used in the long-term treatment of a client whose primary problem is substance abuse. As with other parts of this manual, the scope of an individual client's problems and behaviors may encompass more than is directly addressed in this section; please refer to other care plans as appropriate.

Alcohol is a drug that causes central nervous system depression. With chronic use and abuse, the central nervous system is chronically depressed. An abrupt cessation of drinking, then, causes a rebound hyperactivity of the central nervous system. This produces a variety of withdrawal phenomena. The particular phenomena are peculiar to each client, the client's pattern of use, and the chronicity of excessive intake of alcohol. The most common withdrawal symptoms can be summarized as follows:

1. *Tremors.* Characterized by irritability, rapid pulse, elevated blood pressure, diaphoresis, sleep disturbances, and coarse tremors. Tremors vary from shaky hands to involvement of the entire body.
2. *Alcohol hallucinosis.* Characterized by misperception and misinterpretation of real stimuli in the environment (not to be confused with hallucinations), sleep disturbances, or nightmares. The client remains oriented to person, place, and time.
3. *Seizures.* These are major motor seizures, usually referred to as *grand mal*. Medical treatment is required.
4. *Auditory hallucinations.* These are true hallucinations, but are caused by cessation of alcohol intake rather than a psychiatric disorder such as schizophrenia. The client hears voices, which are usually threatening or ridiculing. These voices may sound familiar to the client— someone he or she knows.
5. *Delirium tremens (DTs).* This is the most serious form of alcohol withdrawal. Twenty percent of all clients who develop DTs die, even with medical treatment. DTs begins with tremors, rapid pulse, fever, and elevated blood pressure. Rather than improving in a few days, the client's condition worsens over time. The client becomes confused, has delusions, and auditory and visual hallucinations (frequently of bugs, snakes, or rodents). The client feels pursued and fearful. DTs may last from 2 to 7 days and may involve physical complications such as pneumonia or cardiac failure.

BEHAVIORS OR PROBLEMS

Restlessness, sleeplessness
Impaired nutritional status
Fluid and electrolyte imbalance
Seizures
Hallucinations (see Care Plan 7, Hallucinations)
Delusions (see Care Plan 6, Delusions)
Confusion
Disorientation
Belligerent, uncooperative behavior
Hostility
Delirium tremens
Physical exhaustion
Additional physical problems such as:
    Liver failure
    Cirrhosis
    Pancreatitis
    Gastrointestinal bleeding
    Esophageal varices
    Renal function impairment
    Ascites
    Dehydration
    Edema in extremities

SHORT-TERM GOALS

Maintain homeostasis and prevent physical complications.
Prevent the client from injuring self or others.
Reorient the client to reality.

LONG-TERM GOALS

Abstain from alcohol and other drugs.
Participate in a substance abuse treatment program.

NURSING OBJECTIVES	NURSING ACTIONS
Maintain homeostasis. Minimize withdrawal symptoms. Promote rest and sleep.	Monitor the client's vital signs, especially pulse and blood pressure. These vital signs will help determine the client's need for medication. Also observe the client for physical symptoms and changes. Alert the physician to any symptoms or changes observed.
	Complete the physical assessment of the client: ask what and how much the client usually drinks, also the time and the amount of his or her last drink.
	Offer fluids frequently, especially juices and malts. Serve only decaffeinated coffee, as caffeine will increase tremors. IV therapy may be indicated in severe withdrawal.
	Monitor the client's fluid and electrolyte balance.
	Administer medication to minimize the withdrawal progression or complications and facilitate sleep.
Prevent injury; provide a safe environment.	Institute seizure precautions, according to hospital policy (e.g., padded tongue blade in room, padded side rails, side rails up at night).
	Provide only an electric shaver for shaving.
	Monitor the client's sleep pattern—he or she may need to be restrained at night if confused and wanders or attempts to climb out of bed.
	See also Care Plan 23, Hostility, and Care Plan 24, Aggressive Behavior.
Improve personal hygiene.	Encourage the client to bathe, wash hair, and wear clean clothes.
	Assist the client as necessary; it may be necessary to provide complete physical care, depending on the severity of the client's withdrawal.
Orient the client to reality.	Reorient the client to person, time, place and situation as needed.

NURSING OBJECTIVES *(Continued)*	NURSING ACTIONS *(Continued)*
	Talk to the client in simple, direct concrete language. Do not try to discuss feelings or plans for treatment or changes in lifestyle when client is intoxicated or in severe withdrawal. This will be a futile effort, frustrating to both you and the client.
Provide emotional support. Increase reality content to decrease delusions or hallucinations.	Reassure the client that bugs, snakes, and so on, are not really there.
	Tell the client that you know these "sights" appear real to him or her and empathize with the fear that the client is experiencing.
	Do not moralize or chastise the client for his or her alcoholism. Maintain a nonjudgmental attitude.
	See also Care Plan 6, Delusions and Care Plan 7, Hallucinations.
Improve nutritional status.	Provide food or nourishing fluids as soon as the client can tolerate eating; have something available at night. (Bland food is usually tolerated best at first.)

Drug Withdrawal

Two characteristics of physiological addiction to drugs are tolerance (the need to increase the dose to achieve the same effect) and withdrawal. Withdrawal symptoms occur at some time after the last dose of the drug and are specific to the type of drug taken. Withdrawal signs and symptoms for the major categories of drugs are as follows:

Opiates: morphine, heroin, Dilaudid, codeine, Demerol. Initially (8 to 12 hours after the last time the drug was taken): perspiration, yawning, lacrimation, rhinorrhea, sneezing. Followed by dilated pupils, anorexia, restlessness, insomnia, nausea, vomiting, diarrhea, chills, abdominal cramps which may last up to 72 hours after last dose. These symptoms then subside over the next 4 to 7 days.

Central nervous system depressants: hypnotics and sedatives. *Note*: Withdrawal can be life-threatening. Initially (10 to 16 hours after the last time the drug was taken): restlessness, anxiety, weakness, irritability, nausea, vomiting, tremors, hyperreflexia. Two to three days after the last time the drug was taken: delirium, fever, seizures. Without medical treatment, death may occur.

Stimulants:
a. *Cocaine*. Depression, lassitude, headache, excessive sleeping.
b. *Amphetamines*. Clients may experience "crash"—the client is paranoid, feels persecuted, may act out physically. Also may exhibit excessive sleepiness, hunger, or thirst.

Clients with drug use or abuse problems may have poor general health, especially in the area of nutrition. These clients are more susceptible to infections, hepatitis, gastrointestinal disturbances, and so forth.

Clients who abuse prescription drugs have the same problems and difficulties as do clients who abuse illicit drugs. Clients who use illicit drugs may have the additional problem of inadvertently taking larger doses or additional substances without knowing it.

Do not ask the client for or even listen if the client attempts to reveal the names or locations of illicit drug sources to you. You do not need this information to work with the client.

BEHAVIORS OR PROBLEMS

Pertaining to all types of drugs:

Anxiety
Fearfulness
Mood alteration
Drastic mood swings (e.g., from elation to anger or crying)
Uncooperative, belligerent behavior
Disturbances of concentration, attention span, or ability to follow directions
Impaired nutritional status
Fluid and electrolyte imbalances
Physical discomfort and symptoms (according to type of drug)
(For withdrawal from alcohol, see Care Plan 17, Alcohol Detoxification.)

SHORT-TERM GOALS

The client will be drug-free.
Maintain homeostasis and prevent or treat physical complications.

Decrease fear, anxiety, or paranoia.
Provide a safe environment.
Prevent injury to the client or others.
Decrease the client's discomfort.

Develop abilities to cope with stress or crises by nonchemical means.
Develop strengths and coping mechanisms necessary to maintain a chemical-free lifestyle.
Develop and maintain significant interpersonal relationships.
Follow-up care or referral to other agencies as necessary or appropriate for occupational, legal, etc., assistance. (See Care Plan 2, Discharge Planning.)

LONG-TERM GOALS

Referral to and participation in a substance abuse treatment program.

NURSING OBJECTIVES	*NURSING ACTIONS*
Determine baseline data regarding the client's drug intake.	Obtain the client's history, including the kind, amount, route, and time of last drug use. Consult the client's family or significant others to obtain or validate the client's information if necessary. *Remember*: the client may maximize or minimize drug use.
	It may be helpful to obtain blood or urine specimens (or both) for drug screening on admission, per the physician's orders.
	Stress that the above information is needed to help treat the client and to make him or her more comfortable and that information obtained by the nurse or the medical staff is not for legal or prosecution purposes.
	Remain nonjudgmental in your approach to the client or his or her significant others.
	Develop a nursing care plan based on information about the client's drug use that is appropriate for the client's physical needs.
Maintain adequate nutrition and hydration.	Monitor the client's intake and output.
	Encourage the taking of fluids orally, especially juice, fortified malts, or milk. If the client is vomiting, IV therapy may be necessary.
	Initiate and encourage the intake of foods as soon as the client can tolerate them.
	Be aware of the client's fluid and electrolyte balance.
	See Care Plan 15, Client Who Will Not Eat.

NURSING OBJECTIVES (Continued)	NURSING ACTIONS (Continued)
Provide a safe environment for the client.	Place the client in a room near the nurses' station or where the staff can observe the client closely.
	It may be necessary to assign a staff member to remain with the client at all times.
	Restraints may be necessary to keep the client from harming self or others.
	See Care Plan 10, Suicidal Behavior.
	Institute seizure precautions as appropriate, according to hospital policy (e.g., padded tongue blade in room, padded side rails, side rails up at night).
Maintain homeostasis; minimize withdrawal symptoms and physical complications. Decrease the client's discomfort.	Be aware of PRN medication orders to decrease physical symptoms. Do not allow the client to be needlessly uncomfortable, but do not use medications too liberally. *Remember*: The client is already experiencing drug effects.
	Monitor and record the client's vital signs frequently (every 15 minutes) until they begin to stabilize. Then check vital signs every 30 minutes, every hour, and so forth, thereafter.
Promote rest and sleep.	Talk with the client quietly in short simple terms. Do not chatter or make social conversation.
	Be comfortable with silence. You may touch or hold the client's hand if these actions comfort or reassure the client.
	Assist the client as necessary; it may be necessary to provide complete physical care, depending on the severity of the withdrawal symptoms.
Provide emotional support.	Do not moralize or chastise the client for his or her substance use/abuse; maintain a nonjudgmental attitude.
	Talk with the client using simple, concrete language. Do not attempt to discuss the client's feelings, plans for treatment, or possible changes in the client's lifestyle while the client is drug-influenced or in acute/severe withdrawal. This will be a futile effort, frustrating to both you and the client.

NURSING OBJECTIVES *(Continued)*	NURSING ACTIONS *(Continued)*
—when the client is confused or disoriented.	Reorient the client to person, time, place, and situation as indicated.
—when the client is irritable, tremulous, or restless.	Decrease environmental stimuli (e.g., bright lights, television, visitors). Avoid lengthy interactions; keep your voice soft; speak clearly.
—when the client is fearful, paranoid, or feels persecuted.	See Care Plan 6, Delusions, and Care Plan 22, Paranoid Client.
—when the client is acting out.	See Care Plan 24, Aggressive Behavior, and Care Plan 23, Hostility.

Substance Abuse Treatment Program

Substance abuse of alcohol or other drugs is an illness. It is not a moral weakness or a lack of will power. Detoxification must first occur for the client to become successfully involved in treatment. It is important to involve the client's significant others in the treatment (whenever possible) to work toward resolving their problems and feelings and facilitate the client's recovery.

The multiple abuse of alcohol and tranquilizers or other drugs is common. It is important that the client does *not* just "transfer substances," that is, the client quits using alcohol, but relies on tranquilizers or "nerve pills" to deal with stressful feelings or situations.

BEHAVIORS OR PROBLEMS

Denial of the illness
Minimizes his or her use of chemical substances
Many somatic complaints
Blames others for problems
Reluctant to talk about self or personal problems
View of self as "different" from others
Veiled anger
Hostility
Self-pity
Rationalization of problems
Use of intellectualization as a defense mechanism
Physical isolation

Superficial relationships
Inability to form and maintain deep personal relationships
Marital or family problems
Financial problems
Employment problems
Personality disorder (see Care Plan 29, Antisocial Behavior) or other psychiatric problems (see Care Plan 9, Depression, Care Plan 10, Suicidal Behavior, and other care plans as appropriate)

SHORT-TERM GOALS

Accept personal responsibility for behavior.
Recognize the negative effects of his or her behavior on others.
Accurately identify and express feelings.
Accept the fact of chemical dependence, and that dependence is an illness.

LONG-TERM GOALS

Develop acceptable alternative methods of dealing with feelings and situations.
Good discharge planning (with opportunity for employment, follow-up support systems, and so forth).
Maintain abstinence from chemical substances.

NURSING OBJECTIVES	NURSING ACTIONS
Focus on problems of substance abuse.	Avoid the client's attempts to focus only on external problems (such as marital, financial, or employment problems) exclusively without relating the problem of substance abuse. The problem of substance abuse must be dealt with first since it affects all other areas.
Dispel myths about chemical abuse.	Provide the client with factual information about substance abuse. Do this in a matter-of-fact, rather than argumentative, manner. Common myths include: "I'm not an alcoholic if I only drink beer or only drink on weekends"; "I can learn to just use drugs socially"; and so forth.
Identify problems in the client's life and their relationship with substance abuse.	Encourage the client to identify behaviors that have caused family difficulties and other problems in his or her life.
	Do not allow the client to rationalize or explain away difficulties or to blame problems on others or on circumstances beyond the client's control.
	Consistently redirect the client's focus to his or her own problems and what the client personally can do about them.
	Encourage all other clients in the program to provide feedback for each other.
	Give positive reinforcement for the client's identification and expression of feelings, and any insight shown into his or her behaviors and consequences.
Develop alternative methods of dealing with stress or conflict.	Encourage the client to explore alternative ways to deal with stress and difficult situations.
	Help the client develop skills in defining problems, planning problem-solving approaches, implementing solutions, and evaluating the process.
	Assist the client to identify and express his or her feelings in acceptable ways and give positive reinforcement.
	Utilize a group of the client and the client's peers to provide confrontation, positive feedback, and the sharing of feelings.

NURSING OBJECTIVES (*Continued*)	*NURSING ACTIONS* (*Continued*)
Direct the client's focus to his or her present situation.	Focus the client's attention on the "here and now" situation—what can the client do *now* to redirect his or her behavior and life?
	Avoid discussion of "unanswerable" questions, for example, *why* the client uses chemicals.
	Assist the client to the conclusion that sobriety is a choice the client can make.
	Assist the client to view life and the quest for sobriety in feasible terms. The client may be overwhelmed by thoughts such as "How can I avoid using chemicals for the rest of my life?" "What can I do today or this week?" is a much more attainable goal. The client needs to believe she or he *can* succeed in order to do so.
Prepare the client for discharge.	See Care Plan 2, Discharge Planning.

Care Plans Related to Other Behaviors or Problems

The behaviors and disorders addressed in this section may occur in concert with various other problems in this and other sections of the manual. Some of these problems may be manifested by a client with a personality disorder (such as anti-social or hysterical behavior) or a neurosis (e.g., obsessive thoughts and compulsive behavior), or as a part of another disorder (e.g., withdrawn behavior). These care plans are especially suited to the process of incorporating specific elements into an individual care plan for a particular client as appropriate, according to the actual behaviors and problems encountered in the assessment of that client.

Transient-Situational Adjustment Reactions

Transient-situational adjustment reactions are usually temporary difficulties that occur when the client is adjusting to changes in his or her life situation or to the new tasks of a particular time in life. These disturbances are classified primarily by the age or period of the client's life as follows:

1. *Childhood*: 3 to 12 years old. The precipitating difficulty is usually adjustment to school, a major geographical move, the death of a parent, or the divorce of parents.
2. *Adolescence*: 13 to 18 years old. Difficulties may include normal adolescent tasks that are temporarily overwhelming, loss of or divorce of parents, graduation from high school, beginning college or employment, or leaving home.
3. *Young adulthood*: 18 to 35 years old. Difficult situations include college graduation, marriage, the birth of children, the death of a spouse or child, a change in career, or divorce.
4. *Middle age*: 35 to 60 years old. Problems include divorce, the death of a spouse or child, children leaving home, the birth of grandchildren, the loss of youth and vitality, menopause, chronic illness, or declining health.
5. *Old age*: 60 years old and above. Problems are primarily the loss of a spouse, retirement, physical health problems, advancing age, or loneliness.

Clients who are experiencing transient-situational adjustment reactions typically cope with day-to-day life effectively, provided there are no major changes in their roles or in the expectations placed on them. However, major life changes or the culmination of several smaller stressors result in the client's inability to deal with the stress or changes. The stresses or changes that precipitate transient situational disturbances are not always "negative" like divorce, death, or loss of a job. The events may also be generally perceived as happy events such as marriage, the birth of a child, and so on.

BEHAVIORS OR PROBLEMS

Imminent or recent change in life status
Feelings of inadequacy to deal with current life situation
Feelings of being overwhelmed
Loss of a significant person, relationship, or comfortable life stage or pattern (see Care Plan 11, Grief Reaction)
Difficulty adapting to change
Feelings of fear, anxiety, or helplessness
Loss of control of life circumstances
Difficulty implementing effective problem-solving strategies

SHORT-TERM GOALS

Build a trust relationship (see Care Plan 1, Building a Trust Relationship).
Identify the difficulties associated with the current life change or stress.
Decrease feelings of fear, anxiety, helplessness, and being overwhelmed.

LONG-TERM GOALS

Successfully resolve the present crisis.
Reestablish or develop the ability to solve problems effectively.
Develop the ability to deal with life changes outside the hospital setting. (See Care Plan 2, Discharge Planning.)

NURSING OBJECTIVES	NURSING ACTIONS
Identify the difficulties associated with the current life change.	Assist the client to identify the specific aspects of the change that the client likes and the aspects that the client dislikes. It may help to put these in written form.
Decrease feelings of fear, anger, or helplessness.	Encourage the client to openly express feelings; give positive feedback for doing so.
Develop or reestablish the ability to solve problems effectively. Develop the ability to deal with life changes outside the hospital setting.	Assist the client to identify his or her strong areas (assets) and areas of difficulty in dealing with problems or changes. Again, have the client make written lists.
	Assist the client to identify past ways of coping or methods of problem-solving that were successful for the client.
	Encourage the client to apply past successful methods of coping to the present situation.
	Encourage the client to work with his or her family or significant others to gain their help in dealing with aspects of the life change.
	See Care Plan 11, Grief Reaction and Care Plan 2, Discharge Planning.

Withdrawn Behavior

Withdrawn behavior that is mild and transitory, that is, a stunned or dazed period following trauma, is thought to be a defense mechanism. This brief period of "emotional shock" allows the individual to rest and gather resources to cope with the trauma, and can be viewed as healthy behavior. Withdrawn behavior can become increasingly severe, however, and interfere with healthy functioning. Total withdrawal that involves a refusal to eat—such as catatonic stupor—can result in death. *Catatonic stupor* is a condition characterized by mutism, no movement initiated by the client, and no food or fluid intake. If there is no treatment, it can lead to coma and death.

BEHAVIORS OR PROBLEMS

When the withdrawn behavior is due to overwhelming stress:

Lack of spontaneity
Apathy
Lackluster appearance
Inattention to grooming and personal hygiene
Decreased or absent verbal communication
Isolation
Lack of awareness of surroundings
Inadequate food or fluid intake
Retention of urine or feces
Decreased motor activity
Fear
Panic

When the withdrawn behavior is due to severe depression, schizophrenia, or psychosis (in addition to those characteristics listed above):

Fetal position—eyes closed, teeth clenched
Incontinence (of urine or feces)
Muteness
Inability or refusal to eat or drink
Hallucinations (see Care Plan 7, Hallucinations)
Delusions (see Care Plan 6, Delusions)
(See also Care Plan 9, Depression)

SHORT-TERM GOALS

Maintain adequate nutrition and fluid balance.
Provide a safe environment.
Increase the client's feeling of security.
Increase the client's interaction with his or her environment and other people.
Increase the client's physical activity.

LONG-TERM GOALS

Develop alternative methods of dealing with stress.
Maintain contact with reality.
Return to the client's home community and independent living situation.

NURSING OBJECTIVES	NURSING ACTIONS
Establish contact and rapport.	Assess the client's current level of functioning and communication and begin to work with the client at that level.
	If the client is completely withdrawn, mute, and in a fetal position:
	—Sit with the client for regularly scheduled periods of time.
	—Tell the client your name, and that you are there to be with him or her.
	—Remain comfortable with periods of silence; do not overload the client with verbalization.
	—Utilize physical touch with the client (e.g., holding hands, laying your hand on his or her shoulder) as the client tolerates. (If the client responds to touch negatively, remove your hand.) Continue attempts to establish physical touch.
	Talk with the client in a soft voice to express your caring and interest in him or her. Continue to do this with the positive expectation of a response from the client.
	Be alert for nonverbal cues from the client; the results will usually not be dramatic, but rather very gradual and subtle in nature (e.g., hand movement, eyes opening).
	Give the client positive feedback for any response and encourage him or her to continue to reach out.
Maintain adequate food and fluid intake, and adequate elimination.	See Care Plan 15, Client Who Will Not Eat.
	Remain with the client during meals.
	Feed the client if necessary.
	Monitor the client's bowel habits; constipation may occur due to decreased food and fluid and decreased motor activity.
Help the client maintain contact with the environment. Provide sensory stimulation.	Encourage or assist the client to spend short periods of time with one other person at first (e.g., sit with one person for 15 minutes of each hour during the day).

NURSING OBJECTIVES (Continued)	NURSING ACTIONS (Continued)
	Ask the client to open his or her eyes and look at you when you are speaking to him or her.
	Use radio or television in the client's room to provide stimulation.
	Avoid allowing the client to isolate himself or herself in the room for long periods of time.
	Gradually increase the amount of time the client spends with others, and the number of people the client is with.
	Assess the client's level of tolerance of stimuli; do not force too much stimulation too fast.
	Talk with the client as though he or she will respond: continue to expect a response and avoid rapid chatter. Allow adequate time for the client to respond, either verbally or physically.
	Refer to other people, objects, the weather, etc., as you interact with the client.
Increase physical activity.	Walk slowly with the client at first. Progress gradually from gross motor activity (walking, gestures with hands) to activities requiring fine motor skills (jigsaw puzzles, writing).
	If the client is immobile (in a fetal position) provide passive range of motion exercises to maintain joint mobility and muscle tone. Turn the client at least every 2 hours if possible; provide skin care and observe for pressure areas and skin breakdown.
Encourage the expression of emotions. Promote a supportive and secure environment.	Encourage the client to express himself or herself nonverbally (e.g., writing, drawing), which is usually less threatening than verbalization at first.
	Then, encourage the client to verbalize about these communications, and progress to more direct verbal communication as the client tolerates. Encourage the client then to ventilate feelings as much as possible.
	Interact on a one-to-one basis initially, then help the client progress to small groups, and larger groups as tolerated.

CARE PLAN 22

Different psychiatric disorders may include paranoia, for example, paranoid schizophrenia, paranoid state, psychotic depression, organic brain syndrome, involutional psychosis, sensory deprivation, sleep deprivation, and substance abuse. Caffeine, especially in large doses, is suspected of contributing to anxiety or paranoid feelings (or both) in some clients.

Many paranoid clients are of at least average or greater intelligence. Paranoid ideation or behaviors may be rooted in an earlier experience of loss, pain, or disappointment, which was denied by the client (unconsciously). The client uses the defense mechanism of projection to ascribe to others the feelings he or she has (as a result of those earlier experiences and denial) and attempts to protect himself or herself with suspiciousness or paranoia.

The client may have extremely low self-esteem or feel very powerless in his or her life, and therefore compensates with grandiose delusions or ideas of reference to bolster self-esteem or to decrease feelings of powerlessness. The delusions may be grandiose (e.g., the client says he or she is a prominent religious or political figure), destructive, or conspiratorial in nature (e.g., groups of persons are watching, following, torturing, or controlling the client). This may involve *ideas of reference*—the client thinks that statements by others or events are due to, controlled by, or specifically meant for him or her (e.g., that a television program was produced to give the client a message).

BEHAVIORS OR PROBLEMS

Lack of trust
Low self-esteem
Suspicion
Fears
Refusal to eat
Hostility, aggression
Delusions, especially grandiose, and of persecution
Ideas of reference
Hallucinations, especially auditory
Other schizophrenic symptoms
Pacing (or other psychomotor disturbance)
Reluctance or refusal to take medications
Suicidal or homicidal ideations
Inability to carry out activities of daily living, responsibilities at home, work, etc.
Impaired relationships with significant others
Social isolation

SHORT-TERM GOALS

Establish a trust relationship.
Decrease suspicion.
Provide adequate nutrition, hydration, and elimination.
Discourage rumination.
Ensure ingestion of medications.
Increase self-esteem.
Decrease or eliminate delusions, hallucinations, ideas of reference, and other psychotic symptoms.
Decrease or eliminate hostility, violence, and aggression.

LONG-TERM GOALS

Eliminate psychotic and paranoid symptoms.
Develop alternative ways to deal with stress, loss, and pain.
Comply with medication regime.

NURSING OBJECTIVES	NURSING ACTIONS
Establish a trust relationship. Decrease or eliminate suspicion. Decrease or eliminate fears.	Introduce yourself on your first approach to the client, and thereafter if necessary to remind the client. Be nonthreatening in all your approaches to the client. Give the client clear information regarding his or her personal safety on the unit, confidentiality, identity and function of staff members, equipment, and so forth. If the client is pacing, walk with the client to converse if necessary. If the client is hallucinating, try to talk with the client in an area of decreased stimuli. Include the client in the formulation of a treatment plan when possible and appropriate. Do not be secretive with the client. Let the client see the notes that you take in interviews. Answer questions honestly with little or no hesitation. Be aware of the client's presence around the nursing station when discussing the client (or other clients). Do not whisper in the presence of the client. (See Care Plan 1, Building a Trust Relationship.)
Assist the client in identifying and ventilating his or her feelings.	If the client fears that personal feelings (such as anger or hatred) will overwhelm him or her or fears losing control, assure the client that the hospital is a protective environment and that the staff will help the client maintain control—that the client will not be "in trouble" for having feelings. Advise the client not to keep weapons at home. Encourage the client to ventilate feelings. Approach the client for interaction at least once per shift (determine the length of interactions by the client's toleration).

	When the client appears to be having feelings, point this out to the client and tell why you think this (e.g., the situation, the client's facial expression or fidgeting); ask for the client's feelings and feedback regarding your analysis.
	Encourage the client to verbalize or express feelings in other outward ways (e.g., physical activity) at the time the client is experiencing them.
	Use limited role playing with the client to elicit the expression of feelings (e.g., "Pretend that I'm your [wife, husband, etc.] . . . what would you like to say to me right now?").
Ensure ingestion of medications.	Give the liquid form of a medication when possible if the client is reluctant to take medication or if there is a question whether the client is ingesting medication.
	Check the client's mouth if necessary after giving p.o. medications (have the client open mouth, raise tongue, etc.).
	Be straightforward and specific with the client when giving information about his or her medications: tell the client the name of the medication and its desired effects (such as, "to help clear your thinking," or "to decrease your fears," or "to make the voices go away").
	Point out to the client that the medications are a part of the treatment plan and that he or she is expected to take them. Ask the client to honestly tell you that he or she has taken medications.
Decrease or eliminate delusions, ideas of reference, hallucinations, rumination, and other psychotic symptoms.	Do not argue with the client about delusions or ideas of reference, but do interject reality when appropriate, and do not give any indication that you believe as the client does (e.g., say "I don't see it that way.").
	Do not joke with the client regarding his or her beliefs.
	Do not enter into political, religious, or other controversial discussions with the client.

NURSING OBJECTIVES (Continued)	NURSING ACTIONS (Continued)
	Encourage the client to discuss topics other than delusions such as home life, family, or school.
	Do not allow the client to ruminate or to ramble on about delusions; if the client refuses to discuss other topics, talk with him or her about his or her *feelings* regarding the delusions, fears, and so forth; if the client refuses to do this, withdraw your attention (state that you intend to return).
	If the client's delusions or ruminations are religious in nature, a referral to the facility chaplain may be indicated (if the chaplain has special education or experience in this area).
	The staff members may need to reassure the client that the origin of his or her fears is internal, that the fears are not based in external reality.
	Observe the client for expression of symptoms, and try to note environmental factors that precipitate or exacerbate symptoms; then try to manipulate the environment to decrease or control these factors (e.g., audio stimuli, other people).
	See also Care Plan 6, Delusions, Care Plan 7, Hallucinations, and Care Plan 3, Schizophrenia.
Decrease or eliminate hostility and aggression.	Search the client's belongings carefully for weapons. If the client has a vehicle at the facility, consider that there may be one or more weapons in it.
	Be calm and nonthreatening in all your approaches to the client; approach the client with a quiet voice; do not surprise the client.
	Observe the client closely for agitation and decrease stimuli or move the client to a less stimulating area or seclusion area if appropriate.
	Observe the client's interactions with his or her visitors. The length, number, or frequency of visits may need to be limited.
	See also Care Plan 23, Hostility, and Care Plan 24, Aggressive Behavior.

NURSING OBJECTIVES (Continued)	NURSING ACTIONS (Continued)
Encourage the client to join the milieu and develop relationships with other clients and staff members.	At first the staff may need to protect the client from the anger he or she may incite in other clients by his or her paranoid behavior or thoughts.
	After the client's initial days on the unit, begin assigning different staff members to the client and encourage other staff members to approach this client for brief interactions.
Decrease isolation from others.	Begin with helping the client make individual contacts (with staff members and other clients); progress to small informal groups, then larger or more formal groups as the client can tolerate.
	Observe the client's interactions with other clients and encourage the development of appropriate relationships with others.
	Give the client support for any interactions and attempts to interact with others.
	Build the client's socialization skills through the above actions, leisure-time counseling, and through the use of other facility and community resources (e.g., occupational or recreational therapy, outpatient social clubs or groups).
	Try to involve the client in activities and tasks that are noncompetitive at first, then help the client progress to larger and more competitive groups as tolerated.
Increase self-esteem.	Help the client to increase self-esteem by demonstrating an honest interest and concern (do not flatter the client or be otherwise dishonest). Support the client for his or her participation in activities, treatment, and interactions. Provide opportunities for the client to perform activities that are easily accomplished or that the client likes to do, and give support for their completion or success.
Provide (encourage) adequate nutrition, hydration, elimination, sleep, and activities of daily living.	Observe the client's eating, drinking, and elimination patterns and assist the client as necessary.
	If the client is overactive or pacing, frequently offer small amounts of juice, milk, or finger foods that can be ingested while walking.

NURSING OBJECTIVES (Continued)	**NURSING ACTIONS** (Continued)
	Observe and assess the client's caffeine intake (record your observations) and limit this if necessary.
	Monitor and assess the client's sleep patterns and prepare him or her for bedtime by decreasing stimuli, giving a backrub (if tolerated), and administering other comfort measures or medications.
	See also Care Plan 15, Client Who Will Not Eat.

Hostility

Be aware of the client's past behavior: What has the client done in the past? What has the client threatened to do? What are the client's own limits for himself or herself?

Much hostility is the result of feelings that are unacceptable to the client, which the client then projects on others, particularly staff members and other authority figures. Often the client is afraid to express anger appropriately, fearing a loss of control.

Be aware of the medications the client is taking. Some medications (e.g., Valium®) may agitate the client or precipitate outbursts of rage by suppressing inhibitions. Also note PRN medication and restraint orders, should they be necessary.

Remember: All anger is not necessarily "hostility," and therefore is not in need of control. A client's anger may be justified and is often a healthy response to circumstances, feelings, or hospitalization itself (i.e., with an accompanying loss of civil rights or dignity). It is important (ideally) to examine with the client his or her feelings and to support the expression of anger when the client expresses it in ways that are not injurious to the client or others (physically or verbally) and are acceptable to the client. The goal of therapy is not to control the client per se, but to protect the client and others from injury and to help the client develop and utilize healthy ways of expressing and dealing with feelings.

It is extremely important to be aware of your own feelings. If you are angry with the client, you may let the client know and explain why, thereby showing the client an appropriate expression of anger. Do *not* react to the client in a hostile or punitive way.

BEHAVIORS OR PROBLEMS

Verbal aggression or abuse
Physical combativeness (see Care Plan 24, Aggressive Behavior)
Agitation
Restlessness (fidgeting, pacing)
Inability to control voice volume (e.g., shouting)
Outbursts of anger or hostility
"Negative attitude," uncooperative
Resistance to hospitalization or treatment program, medications, etc.
Projection of feelings that are unacceptable to the client
Personality disorder (e.g., antisocial personality), behavioral disorder (e.g., manipulative behavior), or other psychiatric problem (e.g., manic-depressive illness) (see other care plans as appropriate)

SHORT-TERM GOALS

Protect the client and others from injury.
Prevent destruction of property.
Verbalize feelings.
Accept feelings such as anger without guilt.

LONG-TERM GOAL

Develop healthy ways to express and deal with anger.

NURSING OBJECTIVES	NURSING ACTIONS
Build a trust relationship.	See Care Plan 1, Building a Trust Relationship.
Decrease the client's hostile behavior; increase the appropriate expression of angry, hostile feelings.	See Care Plan 24, Aggressive Behavior.
	Be consistent, firm, yet gentle.
	Do not argue with the client. Withdraw your attention if necessary.
	Make it clear that you accept the client as a person, but that certain behaviors (be specific with the client) are unacceptable.
	Give the client support and positive feedback for controlling aggression, assuming and fulfilling responsibilities, appropriate expression of angry and hostile feelings, and verbalization of feelings in general.
Increase the client's verbalization of feelings. Increase the client's insight into his or her behavior.	Involve the client in treatment planning as much as possible.
	Discuss with the client what his or her feelings are and different ways to express and deal with them.
	Use role playing and groups (formal and informal) to facilitate the expression of feelings.
	When the client is not agitated, discuss the client's feelings about his or her hostile behavior, past experiences, consequences, etc., in a matter-of-fact manner.
	With the client, identify goals and expectations for verbalization and behavior, pertaining to both inhospital behavior and behavior after discharge. (See Care Plan 2, Discharge Planning.)
Increase the client's ability to control his or her behavior.	Encourage the client to seek out a staff member when he or she is becoming upset or having strong feelings.
	As early as possible in the treatment program, give the client the responsibility for recognizing and appropriately dealing with his or her feelings.
	Expect the client to take responsibility for self and his or her actions; make this expectation clear to the client.

Decrease the resentment that the client has of staff members or the treatment program; increase the client's cooperation.	Involve the client in decision making regarding his or her treatment as much as possible.
	One person may review with the client the reasons for, benefits of, and other aspects of the treatment program, but this should be done only once (may be written).
	Do not argue with the client regarding treatment, rules, expectations, responsibilities, etc.
	Be specific, firm, and consistent regarding expectations of the client; do not make exceptions.
	It may be helpful to have one staff person designated for decision making regarding the client and special circumstances (see Care Plan 25, Passive-Aggressive or Manipulative Behavior, and "Limit-Setting" in Basic Concepts section).
	Withdraw your attention if necessary if the client is verbally or physically abusive; tell the client that you are doing this and that you will give attention for appropriate behavior.
Decrease verbal abuse.	Do not become personally insulted or defensive.
	Remember: It is not necessarily desirable for the client to like you.
	It may help to view this behavior as a loss of control or as projection on the client's part.
	Withdraw your attention (ignore the client) as much as possible at this time.
	Set and keep limits.
	Support others who are targets of the client's abuse (other clients, visitors, staff members), rather than giving attention to the client for his or her abusive behavior.
	Remain calm. Be in control of your behavior and communicate that control. If you are becoming upset, leave the situation in the hands of other staff members if possible.
	Remain aware of your own feelings. It may be helpful if staff members ventilate their feelings

	in a client-care conference or informally to each other privately. Each staff member should try to identify his or her feelings so they are not denied and subsequently acted out with the client.
Decrease outbursts of hostility or aggression.	Watch for a build-up of anxiety or hostility.
	Be aware of and note the situation and progression of events carefully, including the general situation, precipitating factors, ward tension, level of stimuli, degree of structure in the environment, time, staff members present, others present (clients, visitors, therapists).
	Discuss with the client alternative ways of expressing emotions and releasing physical energy or tension.
	Try to make physical activities available on a regular basis and when the client is becoming upset (e.g., running laps in a gymnasium, using a punching bag).
	Encourage the client to develop a regular exercise program and to exercise when he or she feels the need to release tension.

CARE PLAN 24

Be aware of PRN medication and restraint or seclusion orders.

Be familiar with restraint, seclusion, and staff assistance procedures.

Always maintain control of the situation; remain calm; if you do not feel competent in dealing with a situation, obtain assistance (if possible).

Notify the charge nurse and supervisor as soon as possible in a (potentially) aggressive situation; give them pertinent information—your assessment of the situation and needs for help, the client's name, the client's care plan, orders for medication, restraint, and seclusion.

Remember: The client is not in control of himself or herself, and the staff members must provide control until he or she can regain self-control.

Be aware of and work through your own feelings.

Do not overreact to a situation (e.g., if the client does not need to be restrained, do not restrain him or her).

Remain aware of the client's feelings (e.g., fear, dignity) and the client's rights.

Remember reporting and recording procedures: Chart and complete reports carefully, accurately, and promptly. Remain aware of legal considerations.

If a situation progresses to a point beyond the staff's control, the supervisor may decide to seek outside assistance. Should this occur, the nursing staff will turn the situation completely over to them, and the other clients then become the sole nursing responsibility until the crisis is over.

BEHAVIORS OR PROBLEMS

Possible physical acting out (see also Care Plan 23, Hostility)

Destruction of property

Physical danger to self or others

Feelings of hostility, anger, fear

Agitation, restlessness

SHORT-TERM GOALS

Prevent acting out.

Protect other clients.

Staff members will deal with acting out in a safe, therapeutic manner.

Ventilate feelings verbally rather than physically.

Appropriate (nondestructive) expression of fearful, hostile, or angry feelings.

LONG-TERM GOAL

Develop the ability to deal with tension and aggressive feelings in a non–acting-out manner that is safe for self, others, and property.

NURSING OBJECTIVES	*NURSING ACTIONS*
Prevent physical aggression or acting out that can cause danger to the client or others.	Build a trust relationship with this client as soon as possible, ideally well in advance of aggressive episodes. Watch for a building-up of agitation; try to recognize signs of agitation before physical restraint becomes necessary: Increased restlessness Verbal cues Increased motor activity (pacing, tremors) Increased voice volume Decreased frustration tolerance.
Provide a nonthreatening, therapeutic environment.	Decrease environmental stimulation (if the client is feeling threatened, he or she could perceive any stimulus as a threat): Turn stereo or television off or lower the volume Lower the lights Ask other clients, visitors, etc., to leave the area (or the staff member can go with the client to another room).
Provide an outlet for the client's feelings; encourage verbal expression of feelings.	If the client tells you (verbally or nonverbally) that he or she is feeling hostile, aggressive, or destructive, try to help the client express these feelings, verbally or physically (e.g., remain with the client and listen, use communication techniques; or take the client to the gym or outside for physical exercise). Assure the client that you (the staff) will provide control if he or she cannot control himself or herself. *Remember*: The client may be afraid of what he or she may do if he or she begins to express anger. Show that you are in control without competing with the client and without lowering his or her self-esteem.

NURSING OBJECTIVES *(Continued)*	NURSING ACTIONS *(Continued)*
Deal safely and effectively with the client's physical aggression or acting out.	Do not use physical restraints or techniques without sufficient reason.
	Remain aware of the client's body space or territory: do not trap the client (potentially violent persons have a body-buffer zone up to four times larger than that of other persons).
	Allow the client freedom to move around (within safety limits) unless you are trying to restrain him or her.
	Talk with the client in a low, calm voice. You may need to reorient the client: call the client by name, tell the client your name, where you are, etc.
	Tell the client what you are going to do and what you are doing. Use simple, clear, direct speech; repeat if necessary.
	When a decision to subdue or restrain the client has been made, act quickly and cooperatively with other staff members.
	While subduing or restraining the client, talk with other staff members to ensure coordination of effort (e.g., don't attempt to carry the client until you are sure that everyone is ready).
	Do not strike the client.
	Develop consistent techniques; communicate to one another throughout procedures to prevent the client from hurting self and others.
	Do not help to restrain or subdue the client if you are angry (if possible); do not restrain or subdue the client as a punishment.
Provide safe transportation of the client from one area to another (e.g., into seclusion). Obtain additional staff assistance.	Obtain or develop instructions for all staff members in safe techniques for carrying clients, to provide consistency.
	Have someone clear furniture, and so forth, from the area through which you will be carrying the client.

	If time permits, have one staff member quietly contact the supervisor or other units for help; find out what help is available; and give a clear and concise description of the situation and your needs.
	If the need for help is immediate, follow hospital staff assistance plan (use intercom system to page "Code _____," area), then if possible have one staff member meet the additional help at the unit door with necessary information (e.g., the client's name, situation, goal, plan).
Provide for the safety and needs of other clients.	Do not recruit or allow other clients to help in restraining or subduing a client.
	Do not allow the other clients to watch the situation; take them to a different area; involve them in a spontaneous activity.
	Talk with the other clients, especially after the situation is resolved; allow them to ventilate their feelings.
Deal safely with the client who has a weapon.	If you are not properly trained or skilled in this area, do not attempt to intervene. Keep something (like a pillow, mattress, blanket wrapped around arm) between you and the weapon.
	If it is necessary to remove the weapon, try to kick it out of the client's hand (never reach for a knife with your hand).
	Distract the client momentarily to remove the weapon (throw water in the client's face, yell, etc.).
	You may need to summon outside assistance (especially if the client has a gun). When this is done, the total responsibility for decisions and actions is delegated to the outside authorities present.

Passive-Aggressive or Manipulative Behavior

Passive-aggressive behavior is a type of manipulative behavior whereby a client does not express aggressive (angry, resentful, etc.) feelings directly, but denies them and reveals them instead indirectly through behavior. This behavior may be indicative of a personality disorder. Psychological testing may be appropriate. It also may be appropriate to assess the client's motivation to change his or her ways of relating to others and dealing with situations in general. The client may be merely wanting to get out of a bind, crisis, or special situation. Involve the client in care planning if possible.

Remember your professional role. It is neither necessary (nor particularly desirable) for the client to like you personally. It is not your purpose to be a friend to the client, or the client's purpose to be a friend to you.

BEHAVIORS OR PROBLEMS

Denial of problems
Lack of insight
Resistance to therapy: preoccupation with other clients' problems ("playing therapist"), with staff members, or with unit dynamics to avoid dealing with his or her own problems

Inability or refusal to express emotions directly (especially anger)
Manipulation of staff, family, and other clients
Playing one person (staff member or client) against another
Attempts to gain special treatment or privileges
Attention-seeking behavior
Somatic complaints
Intellectualization or rationalization of problems

SHORT-TERM GOALS

Increase insight.
Decrease manipulative behavior.
Increase ability to express feelings.
Increase self-esteem.
Decrease somatic complaints.

LONG-TERM GOALS

Become independent from hospital environment and staff.
Develop mature, nonmanipulative patterns of dealing with people.

NURSING OBJECTIVES	NURSING ACTIONS
Deal effectively with the client who uses passive-aggressive and manipulative behavior in interactions, relationships, and life situations. Decrease the incidence of the above behavior as much as possible, and replace it with more direct and healthy ways of relating.	*Be consistent,* not only with this particular client over time, but also with all the other clients on the unit (e.g., do not insist that this client follow a rule while excusing another client from the same rule).
	State the limits and the behavior you expect from the client—do not debate, argue, rationalize, or bargain with the client. (See also Care Plan 23, Hostility.)

	Enforce all unit and hospital policies or regulations. Point out reasons for not bending the rules without apologizing.
	Be direct and confrontative if necessary (be sure to examine your own feelings—do not react to the client in anger or punitively).
Decrease manipulation of staff members.	Do not discuss yourself, other staff members, or other clients with this client.
	Set limits on the frequency and length of interactions with the client, particularly those with therapists significant to the client. Set definite and limited appointment times (e.g., Thursday, 2:00–2:30 P.M.) with therapists and allow interactions only at those times.
	Do not attempt to be popular, liked, or the "favorite" of this client.
	Do not accept gifts from the client or encourage a personal dependency relationship.
	Withdraw your attention from the client if the client begins saying that you are "the only staff member I can talk to . . ." or "the only one who understands," and so forth; confront the client with the idea that this is not a good situation. Emphasize the importance of the milieu in his or her therapy.
	Discuss the client's perceptions and feelings about being denied special privileges (such as anger, hurt, feelings of desertion or unworthiness); encourage their ventilation and support the expression of those feelings.
Decrease denial of problems.	Discuss the client's problems in relation to being discharged and his or her life at home, rather than in relation to unit dynamics or policies, except to examine how the client's behavior on the unit reflects general behavior patterns in the client's life.
	Discuss the client's behavior with him or her in a nonjudgmental manner, use nonthreatening similar examples.
	Help the client identify the results and the dynamics of his or her behavior and relation-

NURSING OBJECTIVES *(Continued)*	NURSING ACTIONS *(Continued)*
	ships (e.g., say "You seem to be. . . ." or "What effect do you see . . . ?").
Increase effectiveness of therapy.	Emphasize the client's feelings: Encourage the ventilation and expression of feelings rather than intellectualization.
	Be kind but firm with the client. Make it clear that limits and caring are not mutually exclusive: that you set and maintain limits because you care; that the client can feel hurt from someone who cares about him or her; that caring and discipline are not opposites.
	Involve the client in care planning to assess his or her motivation and establish goals, but do not allow the client to dictate the terms of therapy or treatment (e.g., what type of therapy, which therapists, length and frequency of interactions).
	Involve the client in the full treatment program.
Decrease attention-seeking behavior, acting out, and secondary gains.	Withdraw your attention when the client refuses to be involved in activities or other therapies or when the client's behavior is otherwise inappropriate.
Increase healthy and appropriate adult behavior and interactions.	Give attention and support when the client exhibits appropriate behavior—attends activities, expresses feelings, and so forth.
Decrease somatic complaints.	Treat this client as any other within the limits set by the medical staff. Have a physician write orders giving permission for and limits of activities.
	When the client voices a somatic complaint, treat the issue immediately—refer the client to a nurse or physician or treat according to his or her individual care plan.
	Then, tell the client that you will discuss other things (e.g., feelings); do not engage in lengthy conversations about the client's physical complaints or physical condition.
	Observe and note patterns in somatic complaints (Does the client have a headache when he or she is supposed to go to an activity? Or a stomachache when verbally confronted?).

Dependency or Inadequacy

Clients who are very dependent or who lack adequate skills to deal effectively with daily life may be repeatedly admitted to a hospital with varying complaints or precipitating factors. They may report a complex group of problems resulting from inadequate coping with day-to-day life such as legal problems from writing bad checks or a poor job history. These clients may survive outside the hospital adequately until faced with a change or crisis, which precipitates their admission to a hospital. (See Care Plan 20, Transient-Situational Adjustment Reactions, and Care Plan 11, Grief Reaction.) They may be diagnosed as having personality disorders (e.g., passive-dependent, inadequate, passive-aggressive), depression, transient-situational adjustment reactions, or other psychiatric disorders, including suicidal behavior.

Clients who are dependent may rely on a significant other in their lives (the loss of this person could precipitate admission) or on institutions. The client may then transfer his or her dependency needs to a hospital or staff members.

BEHAVIORS OR PROBLEMS

Dependency on others for basic living skills

Inadequate skills for daily living or to meet changes and crises

Feelings of inadequacy, dependency, worthlessness, failure, or hopelessness

Depression (see Care Plan 9, Depression, and Care Plan 11, Grief Reaction)

History of repeated admissions to hospitals

Suicidal behavior, history of suicidal gestures or attempts (see Care Plan 10, Suicidal Behavior)

Manipulative behavior

Anger, hostility (often covert)

Poor judgment

History of or present legal difficulties

Physical symptoms (see Care Plan 13, Hypochondriacal Behavior)

Substance abuse (see Care Plan 19, Substance Abuse Treatment Program)

SHORT-TERM GOALS

Provide a safe environment.

Protect the client from injury.

Minimize attention-seeking behavior, manipulation of staff and others.

Develop or increase insight.

Ventilate feelings, including anger or hostility.

Effectively deal with physical symptoms, substance abuse, legal difficulties, etc.

Ascertain the client's present skills and level of functioning.

Determine the client's optimum level of functioning.

LONG-TERM GOALS

Reach and maintain the optimum level of functioning.

Build adequate daily-living skills.

Establish an outside support system without encouraging undue dependence.

Terminate client-staff relationships.

Eliminate physical symptoms, manipulative behavior, suicidal behavior, chemical abuse, etc.

Establish adequate skills to deal with life changes and crises or determine a plan of action for client to follow if and when these occur. (See Care Plan 2, Discharge Planning.)

NURSING OBJECTIVES	NURSING ACTIONS
Provide a safe environment. Protect the client (and others) from injury.	In your initial assessment of the client, find out if he or she has any history of suicidal behavior or present suicidal ideation or plans.
	You may wish to place the client in a room near the nursing station or where the client can be easily observed; avoid placing the client in a room near the exit, stairwell, etc.
	Closely supervise the client's use of sharp or other potentially dangerous objects.
	(See also Care Plan 10, Suicidal Behavior.)
Minimize attention-seeking behavior and manipulation of the staff and others.	Be consistent with the client. Set and maintain limits regarding behavior, responsibilities, unit rules, etc.
	Give the client support for direct communication and fulfilling unit and personal responsibilities. Withdraw your attention as much as possible if the client acts out.
	It may be helpful in maintaining consistency to assign the responsibility for decisions regarding the client to one staff member.
	Remember: Although the client must feel that the staff members care about him or her as a person (therapeutically), it is not beneficial to the client to have your sympathy or friendship. Do not undermine the client's independence by encouraging dependence on the staff or institution. (See Care Plan 25, Passive-Aggressive or Manipulative Behavior.)
Deal with or resolve physical symptoms, substance abuse, legal problems, etc.	Do *not* assume that physical symptoms are not genuine or that the client is just manipulating or seeking attention.
	The medical staff should investigate each complaint within a certain time period or at a structured time. Then do not give attention for the client's continued conversation about physical complaints. (See Care Plan 13, Hypochondriacal Behavior.)
	Attempt to determine in your initial assessment of the client the extent of the client's substance use or abuse. Interview the client's significant others

NURSING OBJECTIVES (Continued)	NURSING ACTIONS (Continued)
	if necessary. (See Care Plan 19, Substance Abuse Treatment Program.)
	It may be necessary to work with professionals in other disciplines (e.g., social work, law) as they work with the client on his or her legal problems. Again, take care to promote the client's autonomy and development of skills to deal with problems independently. Do not reinforce the client's patterns of dependence on others.
	When talking with the client concerning the above problems, focus on self-responsibility and active approaches that the client can take in his or her life. Avoid reinforcing the client's passivity, feelings of hopelessness, and so forth.
Ascertain the client's present skills and optimum level of functioning.	In your initial assessment and in subsequent conversations, ask for the client's perceptions of his or her skills, level of functioning, and independence.
	Observe how the client functions in various situations on and off the unit: can the client use the telephone? telephone book? how does the client interact with peers? authority figures? how does the client function with regard to structured activities? unstructured time? competitive situations?
	Give the client feedback regarding your observations; involve the client in planning care to work on deficient areas or to use and augment strengths. Together try to arrive at reasonable and realistic goals. Using written lists, priority schedules, timetables, etc., may help to structure the client's tasks. Promote the use of such tools as aids in achieving and maintaining an independent lifestyle.
	Work with other disciplines (e.g., vocational rehabilitation, therapeutic education) for testing of the client and help in specific situations (e.g., job interview training).
Decrease feelings of worthlessness or hopelessness. Increase self-esteem, insight, and independence.	Encourage the client to ventilate his or her feelings, including anger, hostility, worthlessness, or hopelessness. Give the client support for expressing feelings honestly and openly.

	Encourage the client to share his or her feelings with other clients, in small informal groups at first, progressing to larger, more formal groups.
	At first, structure activities with the client that are simple and within the client's present realm of accomplishment. Give positive feedback for tasks completed and responsibilities fulfilled. Progress to more complex tasks or activities as the client is able.
	Support the client's efforts in doing things for self, even if he or she is not always successful.
	Do not flatter the client or be otherwise dishonest. (See Care Plan 9, Depression.)
Establish adequate skills to deal with future life changes or crises.	Beginning with the initial interview, always work toward the goal of the client's discharge and independence from hospital. Reinforce this concept with the client throughout hospitalization.
Establish a support system without encouraging undue dependence.	Rotate the staff members who work with the client to avoid the client's developing dependence on particular staff members. It is not desirable to be the "only one" the client can talk to.
Terminate the client-staff relationships.	Do not give the client staff members' addresses or phone numbers. Do not allow or encourage the client's socializing with staff members or contacting them personally after discharge.
	When necessary, work with other agencies in the community to meet the client's needs. Remember, however, not to undermine the client by unnecessarily encouraging his or her dependence on yet more institutions. Also, these clients may have all but exhausted community resources in the past so work in this area may need special attention.
	Encourage the client to take direct action to meet personal needs in preparation for discharge and support for doing so. Do not help the client unless it is necessary. For example, allow the client to obtain a newspaper (to check want-ads), identify possible jobs or housing, make appointments, arrange transportation, etc., on his or her own as much as possible.

NURSING OBJECTIVES *(Continued)*	NURSING ACTIONS *(Continued)*
	Anticipate the client's future needs and situations with the client before discharge ("What will you do if . . . ?"). It may help to write down specific strategies, people to contact, etc.
	Encourage the client to identify and build a support system outside of and as independent from the hospital as possible. If the client cannot maintain such a level of independence at this time, continued therapy as an outpatient (individual or group therapy) or involvement in a hospital-sponsored social club may be indicated.

Obsessive thoughts are persistent thoughts that are usually troublesome to the client. *Compulsions* are ritualistic behaviors, usually repetitive in nature. Obsessive thoughts and compulsive behaviors are a means of dealing with excessive anxiety; the client engages in repetitive acts to control anxiety and deal with the obsessive thoughts. *Important to note*: Compulsive behavior is a defense that is perceived by the client as necessary to protect himself or herself from anxiety or impulses that are consciously unacceptable. In early treatment, do not prevent the client from performing compulsive acts. Intervention should be limited at first to harmful or dangerous situations or practices. Drawing undue attention to these behaviors will increase the anxiety that the client is feeling. Initial nursing care should allow the client to be undisturbed in performing his or her rituals. Nursing care should reduce anxiety and build self-esteem.

The particular obsessive thoughts and compulsive behaviors may be symbolic of the client's anxieties or conflicts. Many obsessive thoughts are religious or sexual in nature. The obsessive thoughts also may be destructive or delusional (the client may be obsessed with the thought of killing his or her significant other, or may be convinced that he has cancer or that she is pregnant). The client may also be placing rigid standards on self and others that can be unrealistic or unattainable.

Many people have some obsessive thoughts or compulsive behaviors—the client comes to treatment when the thoughts or behaviors impede or inhibit the person's overall ability to function.

BEHAVIORS OR PROBLEMS

Obsessive thoughts (may be destructive or delusional, see Care Plan 6, Delusions)

Compulsive/ritualistic behavior (e.g., washing hands repeatedly)

Difficulty eating or refusal to eat (see Care Plan 15, Client Who Will Not Eat)

Difficulty sleeping

Ambivalence (difficulty making or carrying out decisions)

Disturbances in normal functioning due to obsessions or compulsive behaviors (e.g., loss of job, loss of or alienation from family members, etc.)

Self-mutilation, other physical problems (e.g., damage to skin from too frequent washing)

Aggression toward others (see Care Plan 24, Aggressive Behavior)

Anxiety

Overemphasis on cleanliness and neatness

Rigidity or extremely high standards—cannot tolerate any deviation from standards

Guilt feelings

Fears

Rumination

Low self-esteem

Difficulty or slowness in completing daily living activities or tasks because of ritualistic behavior

SHORT-TERM GOALS

Identify stresses and anxieties.

Ventilate feelings.

Decrease anxiety, fears, guilt, or rumination.

Build self-esteem.

Ensure adequate nutrition, hydration, and elimination.

Promote independence in and completion of daily living activities.

Eliminate aggression or self-mutilation.

Care for existing injuries and other physical needs.

LONG-TERM GOALS

Eliminate the need for obsessive thoughts and compulsive behavior.

Develop alternative ways of dealing with anxiety, stress, life situations, and feelings.

Decrease obsessive thoughts and ritualistic behavior to the point at which the client can function independently (they may never be entirely abolished).

NURSING OBJECTIVES	NURSING ACTIONS
Decrease anxiety, fears, guilt, or rumination.	At first do not attempt to prevent or call attention to the client's compulsive acts: this may result in increased anxiety.
	Encourage the client to verbally identify his or her concerns, life stresses, anxieties, fears, and so forth.
	Encourage the client to ventilate his or her feelings in ways that are acceptable to the client (verbally, through crying, physical activities, etc.).
	If the client is ruminating (e.g., on his or her worthlessness), acknowledge the client's feelings, but then try to direct the interaction in a positive direction (e.g., the client's specific perceptions of why he or she feels this way and possible ways to deal with these feelings). If the client continues to ruminate, withdraw your attention at that time (tell the client that you will discuss other things and state when you will return or when you will be available for interaction again).
	If the client has delusional fears, do not argue with the client about the logic of these fears (see Care Plan 6, Delusions). Acknowledge the client's feelings; interject reality briefly (e.g., "Your tests show that you are not pregnant"), and move on to a concrete subject for conversation.
	At first, allot specific time periods (such as 10 minutes every hour) when the client can focus on his or her obsessive thoughts or ritualistic behaviors, but he or she must attend to other feelings or problems for the rest of the hour. (This will recognize the significance of these thoughts and acts in the client's life, but still allows a focus on other feelings and problems.) Gradually decrease the time allowed (e.g., from 5 minutes per hour, to 5 minutes every 2 hours).

NURSING OBJECTIVES (Continued)	NURSING ACTIONS (Continued)
Decrease or eliminate the obsessions. Decrease or eliminate compulsive behaviors. Decrease ambivalence and the overemphasis on order or cleanliness.	As the client's anxiety decreases (by identifying and ventilating feelings) and as a trust relationship builds, talk with the client about his or her thoughts and behavior, and about the client's feelings regarding them. Help the client identify alternative behaviors and methods for dealing with increased anxiety. Encourage the client to attempt to decrease the frequency of compulsive behaviors gradually. The client (or staff members) may identify a baseline frequency and then keep a record of the decrease. Give the client verbal support for attempts to lessen the need for ritualistic behavior and to decrease its frequency. Talk with the client about other symptoms as appropriate (e.g., ambivalence, frustration, rigidity) as above. Help the client develop satisfactory coping mechanisms to decrease frustration.
Increase self-esteem.	Help the client to increase his or her self-esteem by demonstrating an honest interest and concern (do not flatter the client or be otherwise dishonest). Support the client for participation in activities, treatment, and interactions. Provide opportunities for the client to participate in activities that are easily accomplished or enjoyed by the client.
Maintain adequate nutrition, hydration, elimination, sleep, and normal activities of daily living.	Observe the client's eating, drinking, and elimination patterns and assist the client as necessary (see Care Plan 15, Client Who Will Not Eat). Monitor and assess the client's sleep patterns and prepare him or her for bedtime by decreasing stimuli, giving a backrub, and other comfort measures or medications. The client may need to begin the bedtime routine earlier than is usual. You may need to allow extra time (e.g., get the client up early) or the client may need to be verbally directed to accomplish the normal activities of daily living.
Decrease or eliminate self-mutilation and aggression.	Treat any existing injury (e.g., cream to reddened skin, protection for eyes).

NURSING OBJECTIVES *(Continued)*	NURSING ACTIONS *(Continued)*
	The client may have to be restrained or otherwise protected from self-mutilation.
	See Care Plan 24, Aggressive Behavior.
	Try to substitute physically safe behavior (even if it is compulsive or ritualistic) to decrease harmful acts. If the client is cutting himself or herself, direct him or her toward tearing paper, for example.

Hysterical Behavior

It is best to work with this client within the observation of other staff members. Clients with hysterical behavior may accuse a staff member of improper sexual comments or advances. Therefore it is best to avoid situations where the client could make such claims.

Clients with hysterical behavior may look and act as though they have few problems or none at times. It is easy for staff members to think they could act appropriately "if the client wanted to do so." Actually, the client must learn appropriate behavior. Family or marital counseling may be indicated to effectively deal with the client's problems.

When the client's seductive dress or behavior results in a sexual advance or response from others, the client may be surprised and say that he or she did not expect that to happen.

These clients may exhibit overt physical signs, typically seizure-like activity, blackouts or fainting spells, and dizziness, which have no organic basis. It is important that the client's physical health status is investigated and determined to be sound before hysterical episodes can be effectively dealt with by the staff. Such episodes almost always happen with an audience or at a time when the client is in an unpleasant situation or wishes to avoid an anticipated situation such as a therapy session or activity.

BEHAVIORS OR PROBLEMS

Low self-esteem
Inability to tolerate or deal with stress or conflict
Overt exaggeration or dramatization of emotions

Emotionally labile (may go from crying to giddiness in a few moments)
Low frustration tolerance
Frequent physical complaints without an organic basis
Seductive behavior
Attention-seeking behavior
Manipulative behavior
Poor interpersonal relationships
Shallow emotions
Lack of consideration for others
Suicidal threats or gestures
Angry outbursts or temper tantrums
Dressing in outlandish or seductive clothing
Uses excessive makeup

SHORT-TERM GOALS

Decrease attention-seeking, seductive, and manipulative behavior.
Develop moderation in habits of dress and makeup.
Increase or develop socially appropriate behavior.
Decrease acting-out behavior—temper tantrums, suicidal gestures.

LONG-TERM GOALS

Improve self-image; increase feelings of worthiness.
Improve ability to deal with frustrations.
Develop appropriate methods to express emotions that are neither shallow nor exaggerated.

NURSING OBJECTIVES	NURSING ACTIONS
Establish a working relationship with the client.	Your initial relationship with the client will be based on establishing your consistency and reliability rather than on a discussion of the client's deep feelings.
	Let the client know you will establish limits on acceptable and unacceptable behavior, and will be consistent in enforcing these limits.
	Identify the client's particular behaviors that are causing problems for him or her (e.g., seductive behavior, physical symptoms, suicidal gestures).
Decrease the client's focus on vague physical complaints.	*Remember*: It must be determined that physical complaints or episodes are indeed without an organic basis.
	Initially it may be necessary to give client 10 minutes per shift to discuss physical concerns. Gradually decrease the time until this behavior is totally eliminated.
Decrease secondary gain from physical complaints.	Do not allow the client to avoid frustrating or unpleasant responsibilities or attendance at activities due to physical complaints (see also Care Plan 25, Passive-Aggressive or Manipulative Behavior).
Decrease manipulative attention-seeking behaviors.	Remove the audience or the client from situations in which attention-seeking behaviors occur.
Decrease suicidal gestures.	Identify inappropriate behaviors to the client in a matter-of-fact manner.
Decrease hysterical episodes of physical symptoms.	Withdraw your attention from the client as long as inappropriate behavior continues.
Develop more acceptable methods of seeking attention.	If the client begins destroying property, harming self, or threatening others, it may be necessary to place the client in a safe, secluded environment. Handle the situation swiftly without arguing or chastising the client, giving as little attention to him or her as is possible.
	When the client regains control and ceases the behavior, then attempt to talk with him or her to explore more acceptable ways of handling frustration and expressing feelings.

NURSING OBJECTIVES *(Continued)*	NURSING ACTIONS *(Continued)*
	Give the client positive feedback when he or she expresses himself or herself appropriately or avoids employing previous behaviors when under stress or frustrated.
Eliminate seductive behavior.	Point out inappropriate dress, grooming, or excessive makeup when they occur. Do so privately and without recrimination.
Encourage more appropriate habits of dress and grooming.	Suggest a more moderate yet attractive choice of clothes or application of makeup.
	Give genuine compliments when the client's appearance is suitable.
	Encourage the client's peers to give positive yet genuine feedback for appearance.
	Explore alternative methods of gaining attention, which are not sexual or seductive in nature.
	Give the client an opportunity to discuss his or her difficulties with interpersonal relationships; encourage the client to express feelings.
	Encourage the client to try out alternative behaviors. Assist the client in having short successful social interchanges with others at first, then help the client progress to discussing feelings, problems, and more emotionally charged issues.

Antisocial Behavior

The history of such clients' problems usually begins in grade school with truancy, poor grades, disruptive behavior in class, and fighting with other children.

The client with antisocial behavior may be charming, full of fun, and entertaining on a superficial social level. He or she usually has the abilities to succeed, is of average or above-average intelligence, and meets people well initially and superficially. This client rarely sees himself or herself as having difficulties and usually does not seek help voluntarily, unless it is to avoid unpleasant consequences (e.g., may consent to hospitalization to avoid jail, divorce, debts, etc.).

Success in making changes in this client may be short-lived. The client may return to jail or hospital repeatedly. It may take several years to modify the pattern of behavior to meet long-term goals. Thus, clients with antisocial behavior can be very frustrating for staff members to work with in a hospital setting.

BEHAVIORS OR PROBLEMS

Lack of close relationships with others
Low frustration tolerance
Impulsive behavior
Desire for immediate pleasure or gratification
Inability to postpone gratification
Poor judgment in future planning

Manipulative behavior (see Care Plan 25, Passive-Aggressive or Manipulative Behavior)
Drug or alcohol use/abuse
Conflict with authority
Poor employment record
Difficulty following rules and obeying laws
Lack of feelings of remorse
Failure to learn and change behavior from past experience or punishment
Socially unacceptable behavior
Failure to accept or handle responsibility

SHORT-TERM GOALS

Identify precipitating behaviors or factors that led to hospitalization.
Decrease unacceptable behavior.
Improve impulse control.
Develop ability to delay gratification.
Develop alternative methods of dealing with frustration.

LONG-TERM GOALS

Develop interpersonal relationships with significant others.
Adhere to rules and laws on return to home community.
Obtain and maintain employment with satisfactory work performance.

NURSING OBJECTIVES	NURSING ACTIONS
Identify the behaviors or actions that led to hospitalization.	Encourage the client to discuss the actions that precipitated hospitalization (e.g., debts, marital problems, a law violation).

	Give positive feedback for honesty. The client may try to play the "sick, helpless" role. Honest identification of the reasons for hospitalization are necessary for future behavior change.
Decrease unacceptable behavior. Establish firm, consistent limits on behavior.	Identify behaviors that are unacceptable for the client. These may be general (e.g., stealing others' possessions) or specific (e.g., embarrassing Ms. X by using profane language or telling off-color stories).
	Develop specific consequences for the identified unacceptable behaviors (e.g., the client may not go to gym that day, or have television privileges revoked, etc.). The consequence must deprive the client of something he or she enjoys.
	Avoid any discussion or debate about why the rules or requirements exist. State the requirement or rule in a matter-of-fact manner. The client may attempt to get special concessions or bend the rules "just this once" with numerous reasons, excuses, and justifications. Avoid arguing with the client.
	Avoid discussing another staff member's actions or statements with the client until the other staff member is present.
	Communicate and document in the client's care plan *all* behaviors and consequences in specific terms for all staff members. The client may attempt to gain favor with individual staff members or play one staff member against another (e.g., "Last night the nurse told me I could do that.").
	Be consistent and firm with the care plan. Do not make independent changes in rules or consequences. Any changes should be made by the staff as a group and the new information conveyed to all staff members working with this client. This includes other disciplines as well. (Also, you may designate a primary staff person to be responsible for minor decisions and refer all questions to this person.)
Improve impulse control. Develop the ability to delay gratification.	Inform the client of the consequences of specific behaviors before the behavior occurs.

NURSING OBJECTIVES (Continued)	NURSING ACTIONS (Continued)
	Avoid attempting to coax or convince the client to do the "right thing."
	Provide the consequence immediately after the behavior in a matter-of-fact manner. *Remember:* If you are angry, the client may take advantage of it. It is better to get out of the situation if possible and let someone else handle it.
	Provide immediate positive feedback or reward for acceptable behavior.
	Require gradually longer periods of acceptable behavior to obtain the reward. Inform the client of changes in requirements and rewards as they occur. For example, at first, the client must demonstrate acceptable behavior for 2 hours to earn 1 hour of television time. Gradually, both requirement and reward are increased. The client could progress to 5 days of acceptable behavior and earn a 2-day weekend pass.
Encourage the verbal expression of frustration.	Encourage the client to identify sources of frustration, how he or she dealt with it previously and the unpleasant consequences that resulted.
	Explore alternative, socially and legally acceptable, methods of dealing with the identified frustrations.
	Assist the client to try alternatives as situations arise. Give positive feedback when the client employs alternatives successfully.
Obtain employment. Discharge to the community.	See Care Plan 2, Discharge Planning.
	Include job-seeking, work attendance, paying debts, court appearances, etc., in the client's required acceptable activities before discharge.

Borderline Personality

This client experiences many dissatisfactions in major life areas at different times, but is intermittently capable of moderate moods, acceptable job performance, and the absence of outbursts. The client with these problems does not always require inpatient care, and when hospitalizations do occur, they are usually short. In fact, extended hospitalizations can result in the client's being less functional in daily life.

BEHAVIORS OR PROBLEMS

Impulsive behavior (e.g., overeating, gambling, shoplifting, promiscuity, excessive spending)
Manipulation of others for the client's own needs (see Care Plan 25, Passive-Aggressive or Manipulative Behavior)
Displays of temper
Inability to control anger (see Care Plan 24, Aggressive Behavior)
Uncertainty about identity (such as gender, self-image, career choice, loyalties)
Chronic feelings of boredom or emptiness
Physically self-damaging acts (see Care Plan 10, Suicidal Behavior)
Intolerance of being alone

SHORT-TERM GOALS

Resolve immediate crisis or difficulty.
Develop alternative ways of expressing anger.
Eliminate self-destructive behaviors.

LONG-TERM GOALS

Eliminate need for inpatient hospitalization.
Develop a support group in the client's home environment or community.
Develop impulse control.

NURSING OBJECTIVES	NURSING ACTIONS
Provide a safe environment.	Assess the client's immediate environment, possessions, and hospital room for potentially dangerous objects.
Decrease self-mutilating or suicidal behavior.	Provide adequate supervision while the client is involved in activities, with other clients, or off the unit.
	Treat any self-mutilating act in a matter-of-fact manner. Give or obtain any physical treatment needed, then change the focus away from the act itself and try to interact with the client about how he or she is feeling.
	See Care Plan 10, Suicidal Behavior.

NURSING OBJECTIVES (Continued)	NURSING ACTIONS (Continued)
Decrease displays of temper or acting out. Help the client develop impulse control. Encourage the nondestructive expression of angry feelings.	Encourage the client to express feelings verbally or in other ways that are nondestructive and acceptable to the client (e.g., writing, drawing, physical activity). Withdraw your attention from the client when acting-out behavior occurs; if the behavior is nondestructive, it may be ignored. If intervention is required (e.g., in the event of destructive behavior), take the client to a secluded, physically safe area without delay (see Care Plan 24, Aggressive Behavior). Give the client positive feedback when he or she is able to express anger verbally or in a nondestructive manner.
Help the client increase his or her ability to discuss concerns about self. Decrease feelings of boredom. Help the client establish supportive relationships with others. Decrease manipulation of others.	With the client, establish acceptable limits in relationships. Provide limits for the client if he or she is unable to do so. Do not allow the client to manipulate or take advantage of other clients or visitors (be aware of the client's interactions and intervene when necessary). See Care Plan 25, Passive-Aggressive or Manipulative Behavior. Assist the client to recognize when he or she is feeling bored, and to identify activities which lessen these feelings. It may help to assist the client to structure his or her time with a written schedule. Encourage the client to meet others in his or her community, to begin to make acquaintances, or contact support groups prior to discharge (see Care Plan 2, Discharge Planning). Assist the client to equate manipulation of others with the loss of their company, which in turn results in boredom and loneliness for the client. Encourage the client to express personal feelings or concerns, including identity questions, uncertainties, fears, and so on. Remain nonjudgmental in these discussions and reassure the client that you will not ridicule him or her or take his or her concerns lightly.
Help the client to resolve any immediate crisis in his or her life.	Encourage the client to identify any particular problem or life situation that precipitated hospitalization.

NURSING OBJECTIVES (Continued)	NURSING ACTIONS (Continued)
Minimize the length of the hospital stay.	Assist the client to obtain aid and use resources, such as social services or vocational rehabilitation, as needed and appropriate.
	Help the client to identify his or her strengths realistically, and also identify successful coping behaviors which the client has used in the past. It may help to have the client make a written list. Encourage the client to try to use these coping behaviors in present and future situations.
	Throughout the client's hospitalization discuss discharge planning in a positive manner, beginning with the initial interview or assessment (see Care Plan 2, Discharge Planning).

Glossary

Acting out. Behavior that occurs as a means of expressing one's feelings. It may be acceptable (crying when one is sad) or unacceptable, even destructive (throwing chairs or hitting another person when one is angry).

Attention-seeking behavior. Actions that occur for the primary purpose of gaining another's attention. It is frequently the type of behavior that forces another person to intervene (e.g., asking someone to talk to you because you feel lonely).

Appropriate. Fitting the circumstances, situation, or environment at a given time. For a client in a psychiatric setting, some behaviors may be appropriate at that time, although those same behaviors would be unacceptable in society in general.

Chemical abuse. See **Substance abuse.**

Commitment. The legal detainment of a person without his or her consent, in a facility for mental health treatment. Usually, the person must meet one of the following criteria to be committed: (1) dangerous to self, (2) dangerous to others, (3) incapable of caring for self in a reasonable manner. (Specific laws may vary from state to state.)

Confrontation. Technique of presenting a person with your perception of that person's behavior, or with conflicts you see between what the person says and what he or she does. The goal of confrontation is for the client to gain insight or progress in the problem-solving process. Thus, confrontation should never be done in a punitive or ridiculing manner.

Denial. The unconscious process of putting aside ideas, conflicts, problems, or any source of emotional discomfort. This is sometimes a healthy response, e.g., as a stage in the grief process, to give the person a chance to organize thoughts and align resources to deal with the current crisis. However, if this is a person's only response, or if it is prolonged, it becomes an unhealthy response, a means of avoiding problems, conflicts, which then may be acted out in other, nonproductive ways.

Feedback. Information provided to a person to increase insight, facilitate the problem-solving process, or give an external interpretation of behavior.

Manipulative behavior. Actions designed to influence another person's response. It frequently helps the person avoid the logical consequences of his or her negative actions. See also **Attention-seeking behavior.**

Milieu. Any specific environment, including a group of persons.

Milieu therapy. A group of persons interacting in a given environment, usually with a mental health orientation, with specific goals of problem-solving, improved mental health, and resolution of difficulties achieved by the interaction within the milieu (group).

One-to-one. Specific situation of one client and one nurse (staff member). This may be for the purpose of interaction or for observation, as with **Suicide precautions.**

Open report. A group situation consisting of clients and staff members with participation by all persons. The group functions as a forum for clients to give their perceptions of themselves and each other (that is, to report themselves, rather than to have staff members report on them to each other without the clients' presence). This is usually held at the end of the day or before nursing report and charting.

Optimal level of functioning. The highest level of mental and physical wellness attained by a given individual. This is influenced by the person's inherent capabilities, the environment, coping mechanisms, and internal and external stressors.

Passive-aggressive behavior. A type of manipulative behavior whereby a client does not express aggressive (angry, resentful) feelings directly, but denies them and reveals them instead indirectly through behavior.

Precipitating factor. A situation or factor of importance to the client that is related to the development of an unhealthy response. It may be a major event (e.g., death in family, loss of job) or something that may seem minor to others (e.g., an altercation with a friend). It is important to remember that the client's perception of the magnitude of the event is the most significant factor to assess.

Reinforcement. A consequence to behavior which may be positive (a reward having value to the client designed to perpetuate behavior) or negative (a consequence that the client perceives as negative designed to eliminate or decrease certain behaviors).

Relaxation techniques. Specific techniques to promote physical and mental relaxation, which can be taught by a nurse to a client. These may include breathing exercises (slow, deep, regular conscious breathing), skeletal muscle tensing/relaxing exercises, etc., as well as suggestions for prebedtime measures such as a warm bath or warm milk.

Rumination. Persistent meditation or pondering of thoughts. Carried to excess, rumination over past or present feelings (e.g., worthlessness, guilt) can replace constructive problem-solving.

Secondary gains. Benefits that a client derives from exhibiting certain behaviors or from illness or hospitalization that are not the most direct consequences of that behavior. For example, the client may be successfully avoiding certain responsibilities, receiving attention, or manipulating others as a result of behaviors or illness.

Seizure precautions. Measures taken to ensure the client's safety when and if seizure activity occurs. They generally include padded side rails of bed, airway or padded tongue blade at bedside, and the alerting of staff members to the potential for seizures.

Sheltered setting. An environment in which some special limits exist and some factors are controlled for the specific purpose of protecting clients who are unable to protect themselves adequately at a given time, for example, a hospital, a rehabilitation work environment, a group home, or supervised apartments.

Significant other. A person who is important or valuable to another. This person may be a spouse or relative, but could also be a friend, employer, or roommate.

Substance abuse. The taking of any element into the body to produce a specific effect to the extent that, in time, achieving this effect gains priority over any or all major life concerns. Chemicals (e.g., alcohol, glue, medication) are frequently the elements used. The substance is desired and used even when overall effects to physical or emotional health are deleterious.

Suicidal gesture. A behavior that is self-destructive in nature, but not lethal (for example, writing a suicide note, then taking 10 aspirin tablets). It is usually considered to be manipulative behavior, but may be a result of the client's ignorance of the effects of his or her behavior.

Suicidal ideation. Thoughts of committing suicide or thoughts of methods to commit suicide.

Suicide precautions. Specific actions taken by the nursing staff to protect a client from suicidal gestures and attempts and to ensure close observation of the client.

Support system or group. Persons, organizations, or institutions that provide help and assistance to a person in coping or dealing with problems or life situations, for example, family, friends, Alcoholics Anonymous, Weight Watchers, an out-patient department.

Therapeutic milieu. See **Milieu; Milieu therapy.**

Withdraw attention. Ignoring a client or physically leaving a client alone for the purpose of reducing or eliminating an undesirable behavior or topic of interaction. This is effective only if attention is valuable to that client and if attention is given to the client for desired behaviors.

Bibliography

Clark, C. C. Tactics for counteracting staff apathy and hopelessness on a psychiatric unit. *J. Psychiatr. Nurs.* 13:3, 1975.

Freedman, A. M., Kaplan, H. I., and Sadock, B. J. *Comprehensive Textbook of Psychiatry II* (2nd ed.). Baltimore: Williams & Wilkins, 1975.

Haber, J., et al. *Comprehensive Psychiatric Nursing.* New York: McGraw-Hill, 1978.

Hext, M., and Murchlan, A. Adolescent anoerexia nervosa: The patient; An approach. *J. Psychiatr. Nurs.* 10:18, 1972.

Kalkman, M. E. *Psychiatric Nursing* (3rd ed.). New York: McGraw-Hill, 1967.

Kalkman, M. E., and Davis, A. J. *New Dimensions in Mental Health—Psychiatric Nursing* (5th ed.). New York: McGraw-Hill, 1980.

Kilgalen, R. K. The effective use of seclusion. *J. Psychiatr. Nurs.* 15:22, 1977.

Kinney, J., and Leaton, G. *Loosening the Grip.* St. Louis: Mosby, 1978.

Kyes, J. J., and Hofling, C. K. *Basic Psychiatric Concepts in Nursing* (4th ed.). Philadelphia: Lippincott, 1980.

Lathrop, V. G. Aggression as a response. *Perspect. Psychiatr. Care* 16:202, 1978.

Lenefsky, B., de Palma, T., and Locicero, D. Management of violent behaviors. *Perspect. Psychiatr. Care* 16:212, 1978.

Litwork, E., Weber, R., Rux, J., DeForeest, J., Davies, R. *Considerations in Therapy with Lesbian Clients.* A Symposium presented at the 1978 Midwinter Conference of the Association for Women in Psychology, Pittsburgh, Pa. Philadelphia: Women's Resources, 1979.

Loesch, L. C., and Loesch, N. A. What do you say after you say mm-hmm? *Am. J. Nurs.* 75:807, 1975.

Manfreda, M. L., and Krampitz, S. D. *Psychiatric Nursing* (10th ed.). Philadelphia: F. A. Davis Co., 1977.

Mereness, D. A., and Taylor, C. M. *Essentials of Psychiatric Nursing* (9th ed.). St. Louis: Mosby, 1974.

Robinson, L. *Psychiatric Nursing as a Human Experience* (2nd ed.). Philadelphia: Saunders, 1977.

Schmidt, M. P. W., and Duncan, B. A. B. Modifying eating behavior in anorexia nervosa. *Am. J. Nurs.* 74:1646, 1974.

Solomon, P., and Patch, V. D. (eds.). *Handbook of Psychiatry.* Los Altos, Calif.: Lange Medical Publications, 1969.

Stafford, L. Depression and self-destructive behavior. *J. Psychiatr. Nurs.* 14:37, 1976.

Stewart, A. T. Handling the aggressive patient. *Perspect. Psychiatr. Care* 16:228, 1978.

Stuart, G. W., and Sundeen, S. J. *Principles and Practices of Psychiatric Nursing.* St. Louis: Mosby, 1978.

Ulsafer, J. A relationship of existential philosophy to psychiatric nursing. *Perspect. Psychiatr. Care* 14:23, 1976.

U.S. Bureau of the Census. *Statistical Abstract of the United States: 1979* (100th ed.). Washington, D.C.: 1979. Pp. 76, 79, 176, 181–183, 894.

INDEX

Index